NON-INVASIVE IMAGING OF ATHEROSCLEROSIS

Developments in Cardiovascular Medicine

M.LeWinter. H. Suga and M.W. Watkins (eds.): *Cardiac Energetics: From Emax to Pressure-volume Area.* 1995   ISBN 0-7923-3721-2
R.J. Siegel (ed.): *Ultrasound Angioplasty.* 1995   ISBN 0-7923-3722-0
D.M. Yellon and G.J. Gross (eds.): *Myocardial Protection and the Katp Channel.* 1995
                ISBN 0-7923-3791-3
A.V.G. Bruschke. J.H.C. Reiber. K.I. Lie and H.J.J. Wellens (eds.): *Lipid Lowering Therapy and Progression of Coronary Atherosclerosis.* 1996 ISBN 0-7923-3807-3
A.S.A. Abd-Elfattah and A.S. Wechsler (eds.): *Purines and Myocardial Protection.* 1995
                ISBN 0-7923-3831-6
M. Morad, S. Ebashi, W. Trautwein and Y. Kurachi (eds.): *Molecular Physiology and Pharmacology of Cardiac Ion Channels and Transporters.* 1996 ISBN 0-7923-3913-4
A.M. Oto (ed.): *Practice and Progress in Cardiac Pacing and Electrophysiology.* 1996
                ISBN 0-7923-3950-9
W.H. Birkenhager (ed.): *Practical Management of Hypertension. Second Edition.* 1996
                ISBN 0-7923-3952-5
J.C. Chatham, J.R. Forder and J.H. McNeill(eds.):*The Heart In Diabetes.* 1996
                ISBN 0-7923-4052-3
M. Kroll, M. Lehmann (eds.): *Implantable Cardioverter Defibrillator Therapy: The Engineering-Clinical Interface.* 1996   ISBN 0-7923-4300-X
Lloyd Klein (ed.): *Coronary Stenosis Morphology: Analysis and Implication.*
1996   ISBN 0-7923-9867-X
Johan H.C. Reiber, Ernst E. Van der Wall (eds.): *Cardiovascular Imaging.*
1996   ISBN 0-7923-4109-0
A.-M. Salmasi, A. Strano (eds.): *Angiology in Practice.*   ISBN 0-7923-4143-0
Julio E. Perez, Roberto M. Lang, (eds.): *Echocardiography and Cardiovascular Function: Tools for the Next Decade.* 1996   ISBN 0-7923-9884-X
Keith L. March (ed.): *Gene Transfer in the Cardiovascular System: Experimental Approaches and Therapeutic Implications.* 1997 ISBN 0-7923-9859-9
Anne A. Knowlton (ed.): *Heat Shock Proteins and the Cardiovascular System.*
1997   ISBN 0-7923-9910-2
Richard C. Becker (ed.): *The Textbook of Coronary Thrombosis and Thrombolysis.* 1997
                ISBN 0-7923-9923-4
Robert M. Mentzer, Jr., Masafumi Kitakaze, James M. Downey, Masatsugu Hori, (eds): *Adenosine, Cardioprotection and its Clinical Application*
                ISBN 0-7923-9954-4
Ian Graham, Helga Refsum, Irwin H. Rosenberg, Per Magne Ueland (eds.): *Homocysteine Metabolism: From Basic Science to Clinical Medicine*
                ISBN 0-7923-9983-8
Antoine Lafont, Eric Topol (eds.): *Arterial Remodeling: A Critical Factor in Restenosis.*   1997   ISBN 0-7923-8008-8
Michele Mercuri, David D. McPherson, Hisham Bassiouny, Seymour Glagov (eds.): *Non-Invasive Imaging of Atherosclerosis*   ISBN 0-7923-8036-3

NON-INVASIVE IMAGING OF ATHEROSCLEROSIS

EDITED BY

MICHELE MERCURI, M.D. Ph.D.
DAVID D. MCPHERSON, M.D.
HISHAM BASSIOUNY, M.D.
SEYMOUR GLAGOV, M.D.

Editorial Secretary

CYNTHIA A. SHANE

KLUWER ACADEMIC PUBLISHERS
Boston/Dordrecht/London

Distributors for North America:
Kluwer Academic Publishers
101 Philip Drive
Assinippi Park
Norwell, Massachusetts 02061 USA

Distributors for all other countries:
Kluwer Academic Publishers Group
Distribution Centre
Post Office Box 322
3300 AH Dordrecht, THE NETHERLANDS

Library of Congress Cataloging-in-Publication Data

Non-invasive imaging of atherosclerosis/edited by Michele Mercuri....[et al.].
  P. Cm. -- (Developments in cardiovascular medicine: [DICM 199]
 Includes bibliographical references and index.
 ISBN 0-7923-8036-3 (alk. Paper)
 1. Atherosclerosis--Imaging. I. Mercuri, Michele.   II. Series: Developments in cardiovascular medicine : 199.
 [DNLM: 1. Atherosclerosis--diagnosis. 2. Ultrasonography. W1 DE997VME v. 199 1997 / WG 550 N812 1997]
 RC692.N665 1997
 616.1'360754--dc21
 DNLM/DLC
for Library of Congress   97-37849
                                          CIP

Printed on acid-free paper.

Printed in the United States of America

Table of Contents

PREFACE

Despite the resounding and wishful assertion by Brown and Goldsmith (Heart Attacks: gone with the Century?), cardiovascular diseases are still the number one killer in 3 of 5 continents[2]. Importantly, while medical sciences have made unexpected progresses in the understanding and in successfully reducing cardiovascular death, it is uncertain whether the prevalence of cardiovascular disease will decrease or disappear early in the next century.

Large and important clinical trials[3-5] have provided definitive demonstration that significant reduction of LDL-cholesterol decreases total mortality by 30% and cardiovascular mortality by up to 42%. However, despite an effective LDL cholesterol lowering treatment, 5 of 9 patients with myocardial infarction will still die, and 14 of 21 non fatal myocardial infarctions will not be prevented[3]. While more aggressive management of lipid disorders may improve preventive management of acute ischemia, it is also clear that coronary diseases result from several active and interacting risk factors whose culprit is the unstable atherosclerotic plaque. Therefore, it is unlikely that even the most potent and effective lipid lowering drug will put the issue of atherosclerotic disease mortality at rest. Certainly, this goal is not achievable by simply lowering LDL-cholesterol. A comprehensive therapeutical approach is needed including, but not limited to, changes in the arterial wall, the blood flow, the vasomotor tone, the endothelial function and several different constituents of the blood. Invasive and noninvasive interventional clinical trials have also demonstrated that the morphological characteristics of the atherosclerotic plaque can be modified by treatments targeting cardiovascular risk factors [6-8]. However, regression or stabilization of atherosclerosis is slow and occurs only to a small extent. These changes are interpreted as being only partially compatible with the gains in morbidity and mortality cited above. While this may be a matter of discussion the basic fact is that by targeting linear, superficial or volumetric morphologic changes, we are addressing only one side of the problem. An integrated imaging approach including the study of morphology, flow, molecular and mechanical activities of the arterial wall is required.

This book is intended as a primer, reference and review of some of the key features of current activities in the field of atherosclerosis. The principal goal of the editors is to provide material and stimulating ideas to basic scientists and clinical researchers to extend the application of vascular imaging and to further develop methods suitable for investigation of the arterial wall.

Drs. Hisham Bassiouny and Seymour Glagov's section will present and bridge current knowledge about pathology, vascular mechanics and compensatory mechanisms active during atherogenesis. It will explore the early lesion, complications of plaques and early detection of plaques. The section is to provide information to better understand and implement clinical strategies to address plaque growth and plaque instability, and how techniques to detect and monitor atheroma progression must take into account evolutionary biologic changes in atheroma.

The second section, edited by Dr. Michele Mercuri, will review several key methodological issues of B-mode ultrasound imaging and some of the most current data. Quantitative B-mode ultrasound is an established non-invasive tool widely used in large epidemiologic studies and interventional clinical trials of peripheral atherosclerosis. B-mode ultrasound protocols are extremely sophisticated research tools for identifying and weighing new cardiovascular risk factors and assess the efficacy of hypolipidemic and antihypertensive drugs on the arterial wall. The next challenge for B-mode ultrasound will be to demonstrate its predictive power when used at the individual patient level.

In the final section, Dr. McPherson has assembled 3 chapters addressing the most promising areas of development in vascular imaging. This involves new techniques to evaluate the atherosclerotic bed, follow atheroma progression/regression and techniques to evaluate vascular mechanics in atherosclerotic arteries.

Finally, Dr. Randal J. Thomas' chapter provides the book summary and places the application of non-invasive imaging in perspective.

Overall, this book can be used as a methodologic or reference text for all investigators involved in the non-invasive evaluation of atherosclerosis.

We would like to thank *Bonnie J. Kane and Melissa Ramondetta* for their technical advice.

We would like to acknowledge the contribution of Novartis for the publication of the color plate section of this book.

References

1. Brown MS and Goldstein JL: Heart Attacks: Gone with the Century? Science 1996;272:626.
2. American Heart Association: Heart and Stroke Facts: 1996 Statistical Supplement. Dallas, TX, 1996, p.8.
3. Scandinavian Simvastatin Survival Study Group, Baseline Serum Cholesterol and Treatment Effect in the Scandinavian Simvastatin Survival Study (4S). Lancet 1995; 345:1274-1275.
4. Shepherd J, Cobbe SM, Ford I et al. For the West of Scotland Coronary Prevention Study Group. Prevention of Coronary Heart Disease With Pravastatin in Men with Hypercholesterolemia. N Engl J Med 1995; 333:1301-7.
5. Sacks FM, Pfeffer MA, Moye LA et al. For the Cholesterol and Recurrent Events Trial Investigators: The Effects of Pravastatin on Coronary Events After Myocardial Infarction in Patients with Average Cholesterol Levels. N Engl J Med 1996 ; 335-1001- 9.
6. Brown BG, Zhao XQ, Sacco DE, Albers JJ: Lipid lowering and Plaque Regression: New Insights Into Prevention of Plaque Disruption and Clinical Events in Coronary Disease. Circulation 1993; 87:1781-1791.
7. Furberg CD, Adams HP Jr, Applegate WB et al. For the Asymptomatic Carotid Artery Progression Study (ACAPS) Research Group. Effects of Lovastatin on Early Carotid Atherosclerosis and Cardiovascular Events. Circulation 1994; 90:1676-1687.
8. Mercuri M, Bond MG, Sirtori CR et al.: Pravastatin Reduces Carotid Intima Media Thickness Progression in an Asymptomatic Hypercholesterolemia Mediterranean population. The Caroid Atherosclerosis Italian Ultrasound Study. Am J Med 01: 627-634.

CONTRIBUTING AUTHORS

Juan J. Badimon, Ph.D.
Associate Professor of Medicine
Division of Cardiology
Mount Sinai School of Medicine
The Mount Sinai Medical Center
New York, New York
USA

Lina Badimon, Ph.D.
Professor of Medicine
Director of the Cardiovascular
Research Center
Unidad Cardiovascular C.I.D./C.S.I.S.
Laboratory Investigation
Cardiovascular
Barcelona, Spain

Hisham Bassiouny, M.D.
Associate Professor
Departments of Pathology
  and Surgery
University of Chicago
Chicago, Illinois
USA

M. Gene Bond, Ph.D.
Professor
Department of Neurobiology and
Anatomy and the Center for Medical
  Ultrasound
Bowman Gray School of Medicine
  of Wake Forest University
Winston-Salem, North Carolina
USA

Michiel L. Bots, M.D., Ph.D.
Assistant Professor of Epidemiology
Julius Center for Patient Oriented
  Research
Utrecht University Medical School
Utrecht
The Netherlands

Kishnan B. Chandran, Ph.D.
Professor of Biomedical and
Mechanical Engineering
University of Iowa
College of Engineering
Iowa City, Iowa
USA

James H. Chesebro, M.D.
Professor of Medicine
Director of Clinical Research
Cardiovascular Institute
Mount Sinai Medical Center
New York, New York
USA

Valentin Fuster, M.D., Ph.D.
Professor of Medicine
Director, Cardiovascular Institute
Dean of Academic Affairs
Mount Sinai Medical Center
New York, New York
USA

Richard Gallo, M.D.
Interventional Cardiologist
Assistant Professor of Medicine
Montreal Heart Institute
University of Montreal
Montreal, Canada

Seymour Glagov, M.D.
Professor Emeritus
Departments of Pathology
  and Surgery
University of Chicago
Chicago, Illinois
USA

xvi

Diederick E. Grobbee, M.D., Ph.D.
Professor of Clinical Epidemiology
Julius Center for Patient Oriented
  Research
Utrecht University Medical School
Utrecht
The Netherlands

Gregory Lanza, M.D., Ph.D.
Barnes Jewish North Campus
Cardiology Division
St. Louis, Missouri
USA

David D. McPherson, M.D.
Professor of Medicine
Division of Cardiology
Department of Medicine
Northwestern University Medical
  School
Chicago, Illinois
USA

Michele Mercuri, M.D., Ph.D.
Adjunct Associate Professor
Division of Vascular Ultrasound
  Research
Bowman Gray School of Medicine of
Wake Forest University
Winston Salem, North Carolina
USA

James Miller, M.D.
Cardiovascular Division
Washington University School of
  Medicine
Barnes-Jewish Hospital North
St. Louis, Missouri
USA

Rong Tang, M.D.
Research Assistant Professor
Division of Vascular Ultrasound
  Research
Department of Neurobiology and
Anatomy and the Center for Medical
  Ultrasound
Bowman Gray School of Medicine
  of Wake Forest University
Winston-Salem, North Carolina
USA

Randal J. Thomas, M.D.
Associate Professor of Medicine
University of South Carolina School of
  Medicine
Director, Preventive Cardiology
Associate Director, Internal Medicine
Greenville Hospital System
Greenville, South Carolina
USA

Michael J. Vonesh, Ph.D.
Division of Cardiology
Northwestern University Medical
  School
        and
W. L. Gore & Associates
Medical Products Division
Flagstaff, Arizona
USA

Samuel A. Wickline, M.D.
Professor of Medicine
Cardiovascular Division
Washington University School of
  Medicine
Barnes-Jewish Hospital North
St. Louis, Missouri
USA

SECTION I

PATHOLOGY OF ATHEROSCLEROSIS

CAROTID ATHEROSCLEROSIS:
FROM INDUCTION TO COMPLICATION

*Hisham Bassiouny, M.D., F.A.C.S., *Yasuhiro Sakaguchi, M.D.
and Seymour Glagov, M.D.*

*The Departments of Surgery and Pathology
The University of Chicago
Chicago, Illinois U.S.A.
*Nara Medical University
Nara, Japan*

Contents

I. INTRODUCTION

It is estimated that approximately 40 - 50% of cerebrovascular events are related to embolic debris and thrombi originating from atherosclerotic plaque involving the carotid bifurcation. In recent years investigations have focused on better understanding of the pathobiology of plaque formation at the carotid bifurcation and its natural history. Knowledge regarding the role of hemodynamic forces and geometric transitions in the induction and localization of early asymptomatic carotid intimal media thickness has aided in refining evaluation of this region by noninvasive imaging techniques such as B-mode ultrasound. This has permitted study of intima media thickness progression or regression in relation to, and modifications of patients risk profiles.

Sequential changes in plaque size and composition are associated with adaptive configurational and structural changes in the vessel wall which tend to preserve lumen size and contour. These adaptive responses may limit the value of conventional arteriography in quantitation of plaque burden. Other imaging modalities which assess mural structure and composition such as high resolution, transcutaneous or intravascular ultrasound will hopefully better evaluate plaque progression and transition to complex and/or complicated lesions.

Critically stenotic carotid plaques are morphologically complex. The clinical recognition and detection of those morphologic features which connote plaque instability, and predisposition to disruption and symptoms is a desired goal. Insight into these microanatomic features can be studied by detailed examination of excised endarterectomy plaques as symptomatic and asymptomatic patients. Improvements in the resolution of current imaging modalities complemented by three-dimensional image reconstruction are likely to permit more precise evaluation of *in vivo* plaque structure and help in the identification of patients at risk for cerebrovascular events.

In this monograph our current understanding of the pathogenesis of non-occlusive intimal thickening, the adaptive response to developing plaque and the morphologic features underlying or associated with plaque rupture and symptoms are discussed.

II. PATHOGENESIS OF CAROTID ATHEROSCLEROSIS

The pathogenesis of the carotid atherosclerosis has been inferred from observations into the morphology of human plaques, [1-3] from the study of experimental animals models, and from the reactions of artery cells in culture. Recent increased attention to the geometric, microanatomic (artery wall), and mechanical (hemodynamic) microenvironment in which human plaques develop has added significant insights into the tissue processes associated with artery reactions and adaptations to plaque formation and to questions dealing with plaque stability.[4-6, 2] The sequence of events leading to plaque formation is complex and probably variable in relation to the degree and duration of exposure to each of the clinical risk factors and more than likely include the interaction of several processes. Evidence is now abundant that the endothelial cell is not merely a protective barrier against thrombus formation. Endothelial cells are active mediators of many aspects of artery wall function. It is also now clear that the initiating events in plaque formation are not precipitated by focal ulcerations of the lumen surface or by desquamations of endothelial cells.[7] Instead, focal activation of endothelial cells by circulating vasoactive and/or toxic materials engender modifications of endothelial reactivity and metabolism.[8] These result in alterations of permeability, in oxidative modification of the LDL particle, in the liberation of chemoattractants, mitogens, and growth factors that determine migration and proliferation of smooth muscle cells, expression of surface adhesion molecules for leukocytes, disturbances of the antithrombogenic function as well as of factors such as nitric oxide and endothelin-1, which regulate smooth muscle tone in the underlying media. These modifications are reflected in the early intimal lesion in the form of lipid accumulation both in extracellular interstices and within both macrophages and smooth muscle cells in the form of foam cells.[2] Smooth muscle cell accumulation and fibrogenesis are prominent features. In addition to smooth muscle cells, macrophages, and lymphocytes also participate in lesion formation and in the modification of plaque composition by elaboration of growth factors, cytokines, and proteolytic enzymes. These features, as well as evidence of cell necrosis, apoptosis, and stratification of lesion components, indicate that both destructive and defensive modeling healing processes are occurring.

Plaques tend to develop in locations where wall shear stress is relatively low and changes direction in the course of the cardiac cycle.[9, 10] In model studies[11] as well as in color Doppler images in humans (Figure 1, color plate 1), such regions are demonstrably sites of increased residence time for circulating particles; that is, particles tend to remain in these regions over several cardiac cycles, exposing such sites to increased contact with atherogenic agents compared with regions where wall shear stress is elevated and unidirectional. Because flow reversal at such regions occurs during the downstroke of systole, increased heart rate over time is likely to be an additional indirect clinical risk factor for plaque induction.[12, 13]

III. MECHANICAL DETERMINANTS OF NON-ATHEROSCLEROTIC INTIMAL THICKENING: IMPLICATIONS FOR THE DETECTION OF MINIMAL LESIONS AT THE CAROTID BIFURCATION

Artery wall stability depends on the maintenance of normal or otherwise acceptable levels of wall shear stress and tensile stress. Wall shear stress is a direct function of blood flow and viscosity and varies inversely with the third power of the radius. When flow is increased chronically, artery radius increases until the original baseline wall shear stress is restored. For mammalian arteries this value is approximately 15 dynes/cm.[2,14,15,16] When flow is decreased the radius decreases also resulting in restoration of baseline wall shear stress. As regards tensile stress, artery wall thickness is determined by blood pressure and artery radius in accordance with the law of LaPlace. In simplified form, for arteries with thin walls compared to radius, wall tension is proportional to the product of pressure and radius and tensile stress is equal to wall tension divided by the wall thickness. In mammalian development, the thickness of the walls of homologous arteries of similar structure is proportional to the wall tension such that tensile stress is maintained at a baseline level. In the event of reduced flow, and therefore of reduced wall shear stress, thickening of the intima may serve to narrow the lumen, thereby increasing flow and restoring baseline wall shear stress. In the event of adjustments to chronically increased flow, the increased radius results in an increase in wall tension. Tensile stress may be restored to baseline levels or to levels consistent with wall stability by thickening of the wall and/or by changes in structure and composition of the media. There is evidence however, both from animal experimental models[19] and from human vessels[20-22] that the intima may participate in these adaptations. Several studies of the localization of non-atherosclerotic as well as atherosclerotic intimal thickenings in human arteries indicate that both of these types of thickening occur preferentially at locations of reduced and oscillating wall shear stress.[20, 23] These conditions prevail, for example, at the inlet side of aortic branch ostia,[24] the inner curvature at bends, in a somewhat helical distribution, but mainly opposite the flow divider in the internal carotid artery at the carotid bifurcation and in the left main coronary artery opposite the flow divider at the origin of the left circumflex coronary artery.[25]   It has also been proposed that selective locations of intimal thickening are also regions of tensile stress concentration.[26] Just as the complement of media layers of homologous vessels may be related to tensile stress, quantitative evidence has been presented that the layering of non-atherosclerotic intimal thickening may be related to tensile stresses.[22, 27]

Detection of early plaque formation at the carotid bifurcation usually depends on ultrasound measurements of artery wall intima media thickness, ie, IMT,[7] and, in more recent investigations, of corresponding changes in mural mechanical properties. Because of the usual focal and eccentric location of sites of reactive intimal thickening and plaque initiation at the carotid bifurcation in relation to geometric transitions,[8,9] the selection of precise regions to be interrogated is critical. The distribution of early IMT or plaques in this location tends to be helical,[10] in keeping with the flow field (Figure 2). Modifications of this pattern may differ in relation to individual geometric variations. Thus, any single axial location and direction of examination by ultrasound may not identify the site of maximal intimal thickening. The carotid bifurcation is therefore best examined over a range of incident angles and axial locations whenever possible. The role of calcification in defining the extent early carotid atherosclerosis remains to be defined.[11,12]

A possible confounding problem in relating absolute values of IMT to atherogenesis derives from the usual relationships between wall thickness and artery diameter. Media thickness and composition are determined by wall tension for normal homologous vessels in mammals, as well as for specific vessel segments and branches.[14] In addition, both nonatherosclerotic intimal thickening and atherosclerotic plaques may contribute to tensile support as wall tension increases with increased diameter.[15] Thus, it may be appropriate to normalize IMT for early plaque detection in relation to diameter for any given individual and location, particularly if such data are used for epidemiologic comparisons of absolute thickness in relation to risk factors. Such considerations may, however, also be appropriate for sequential studies, for early plaque formation at the carotid bifurcation has been shown to result in artery enlargement[15] and thereby to alterations in tensile stress distribution.

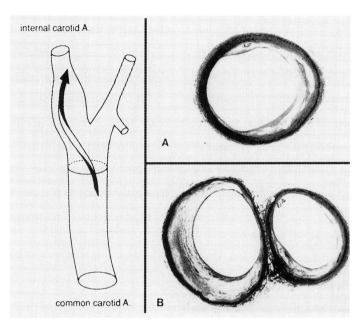

Figure 2. Intimal thickening at the carotid bifurcation, including atherosclerotic plaque formation, follows a helical distribution corresponding to the usual flow pattern in this region. (a) Diagrammatic representation of intimal thickening or plaque distribution, on the flow divider side in the common carotid artery at a distance from the bifurcation and at the far wall opposite the flow divider in the common carotid artery just proximal to the bifurcation and in the proximal internal carotid artery. (b) Section of the common carotid artery at a distance from the bifurcation. The plaque is primarily at the flow divider side. (c) (Section) through the bifurcation at the level of the sinus. Both the internal carotid (larger vessel on the left) and external carotid branches are shown. At this level the plaque is mainly at the far wall opposite the flow divider with somewhat lesser involvement at the anterior and posterior walls. (Adapted from[21] by the kind permission of Elsevier Science Ireland).

IV. ATHEROSCLEROTIC INTIMAL THICKENING

The tendency for investigators to consider any form of intimal thickening to be atherosclerotic or preatherosclerotic, either in experimental animal material or in human arteries, has introduced confusion in relation to the pathogenesis and to the descriptive nomenclature of atherosclerotic lesions and intimal thickenings. The *sine qua non* of atherogenesis as defined in recent deliberations of the Committee on Lesions of the Council on Arteriosclerosis of the American Heart Association[28,29]   is expansion of the intima by the ingress and accumulation of lipoproteins and the subsequent cellular and biosynthetic reactions associated with this accumulation. The reactions include the production and accumulation of fibrocellular matrix components with or without calcification and eventually with or without the presence of lipid. Detailed morphologic studies of lesions from individuals of different age have permitted the establishment of a putative sequence varying from an initial or initiating induction phase to the advanced plaque. Some of the stages in the sequence have characteristic features which may be reflected in imaging studies.

A.   Stages of Atherosclerotic Lesions

Features of early plaque formation are often noted within or upon adaptive intimal thickenings, but these reactive changes are not necessarily or inevitably associated with the induction of atherosclerotic lesions.   Nevertheless, the adaptive thickenings and/or mechanical conditions which prevail at sites of predilection may predispose to the formation of atherosclerotic lesions. In model flow studies of the carotid bifurcation low wall shear stress and the reversal in direction of wall shear during the cardiac cycle results in a delay in clearance of circulating particles from lesion prone regions.[30] Several pulsatile cycles are required to clear circulating particles from the region opposite the flow divider of the proximal internal carotid branch, i.e. a preferential location of lesion formation.[20,23] Regions of low shear and increased particle residence time are likely to be sites of extended exposure to circulating atherogenic agents. The flow divider side is usually spared; in this region wall shear is relatively high, flow remains unidirectional and circulating particles are largely cleared with each pulsatile cycle.[30] Furthermore, reactive intimal thickening in lesion prone regions may delay transmural transport while collagen fibers in intimal thickenings may trap atherogenic lipid particles.[31]

The initial atherosclerotic lesion is characterized by a focal eccentric accumulation of lipid in the intima with intracellular lipid discernible mainly in macrophages (Figure 3, color plate 1). Matrix production is minimal and the lesion is usually not apparent to the unaided eye on gross inspection of the lumen surface without the use of special stains, nor is it likely to be detectable on usual imaging studies. With increased lipid accumulation, lipid is apparent in both macrophages and smooth muscle cells. The advent of smooth muscle cells and matrix fibers along with increased cellularity and lipid accumulation corresponds to the *fatty streak* (or fatty dot or patch) which is visible to the unaided eye without special staining and, depending mainly on lesion thickness, may be revealed by imaging techniques which are sufficiently sensitive to distinguish between the radiologic and sonically lucent fatty streak and the more dense and compact underlying media or intimal adaptive reaction.

In subsequent stages the intima is sufficiently thickened to be readily visualized on images as intima-media thickening or more specifically by techniques which can identify boundaries between lumen and intima and between intima and media. At this stage the fatty streak or patch becomes the lesion type which has been termed the *preatheroma*. Multiple extra-cellular lipid pools are discernable and matrix production is usually more pronounced. Collagen and some elastin fibers accumulate beneath the endothelium and adjacent to the underlying media deep to the lipid pools. Both the subendothelial and juxta-medial fibrous regions are increasingly dense as the lipid pools coalesce to form a distinct lipid core (Figure 4, color plate 2). The subendothelial zone may subsequently become increasingly organized to form a structure, the *fibrous cap*, which tends to resemble the uninvolved media opposite the lesion in both structure and thickness and is usually devoid of either lipid or macrophages. The component cells of the fibrous cap are mainly smooth muscle and tend to be arranged in layers along with similarly oriented collagen and elastin fibers. Changes in the media adjacent to the deep portions of the lesion include evidence of fibrosis which may merge with similar connective tissue changes in the plaque. Alternately, erosion of the media occurs, particularly when the discrete lipid pools coalesce to form a *lipid core* and where the core is located in direct apposition to the media. Coalescence of the lipid pools into a lipid core is accompanied by other evidences of destructive disorganization of the intima and this lesion type has then been termed an *atheroma*. The fibrous reaction becomes increasingly manifest, reinforcing the stratification of the lesion due to the prominence of fibrous tissue in both deep and superficial layers and the associated localization of the lipid core between the fibrous regions. This type of lesion may be termed a *fibroatheroma*.

The lesion may be progress and become increasingly complex in both structure and composition as continued injury, healing and structural modelling and remodeling proceed. Degenerative tissue changes such as dystrophic calcification may become increasingly apparent. The process is continuously modulated by the intensity and duration of exposure to clinical risk factors, and in relation to individual differences in tissue response and local mechanical stresses. Increasingly complex lesions then consist of juxtaposed regions of contrasting composition and therefore of contrasting mechanical properties (Figure 5, color plate 2). Modelling processes such as those which determine the intimal adaptive-reactive responses outlined above continue in relation to the distribution of mechanical stresses within the lesion. Plaques therefore tend to remain stratified usually with the subendothelial fibrocellular reaction and the deeper fibrous reaction persisting. The lumen tends to remain circular or somewhat oval despite a frequent marked deviation from circularity of the outside contour of the vessel.

B.   Arterial Adaptive Response to Developing Plaque

As a plaque enlarges, the artery usually enlarges often preserving a patent and adequate lumen despite the presence of a large and advance, complex lesion.[32,33] The nature of this compensatory reaction is not entirely clear but is closely associated with outward bulging of the artery wall beneath[32,34] the evolving plaque (Figure 6). This effect is noted at nearly all stages of plaque formation and the uninvolved wall opposite the plaque may remain largely unchanged. As with the formation of atherosclerosis-related aneurysms, the changing wall contour beneath the plaque is in all likelihood the result of erosion by metalloproteinases liberated from smooth muscle cells and/or macrophages and accumulated in the lipid core.[35] The limits of compensatory enlargement and outward bulging beneath the lesion may be related to progression of plaque density and rigidity and resistance to proteolysis related to changes in plaque and wall composition and to calcification.

Thus, several morphologic manifestations of putative artery defense against the development of stenosis and flow instability are noted as plaques progress. The lumen tends to remain circular and of regular contour as the eccentric lesion is effectively sequestered by fibrosis and outward bulging of the underlying artery wall.

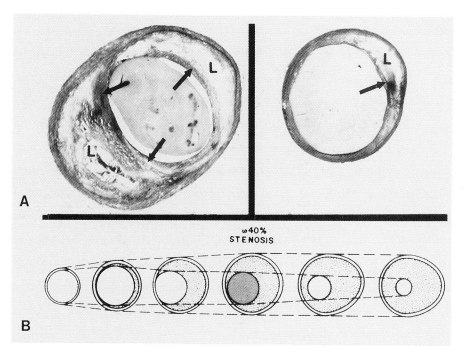

Figure 6.   In relation to the modeling and remodeling processes described, arteries appear to enlarge initially as plaques form, tending to preserve a lumen in adequate cross-section even in the presence of relatively large intimal plaques (32,33).   A, Postmortem sections of the left anterior descending coronary artery taken at the same level in two individuals. The lumen cross-sectional area (L) is approximately the same for each individual, although the lesion area is vastly different. If the artery on the left had to enlarged to compensate for the large plaque that formed, the lumen would have been totally occluded. That artery enlargement is a consequence of plaque formation is indicated by the fact that in any given artery segment lumen cross-sectional area is often similar for involved and uninvolved segments. Enlargement usually occurs only where plaques are forming. B, Diagram of artery (32). Although plaque formation may be arrested at any stage, lumen stenosis appears to be evidence on the average when 40% ore more of the potential lumen area (as defined by the area encompassed by internal elastic lamina), is occupied by plaque. Plaque enlargement is mainly associated with outward bulging of the artery wall beneath the lesion.   (Adapted from Glagov and coworkers (32); with permission).

The fibrous cap isolates the lesion from the circulation and its structure suggests an adaptive modelling reaction which results in what appears to be the neoformation of a supportive media-like structure. Both the outward compensatory bulging process and possibly flow related processes which may cause dilation of the preserved wall opposite the plaque tend to preserve an adequate lumen in the face of advancing disease.

The sequence of morphologic features set forth above are an idealized representation of the characteristic intimal changes associated with plaque formation. It should be noted however that deviations and modifications of these transitions are frequent. Atherosclerotic lesions may stabilize and persist with little subsequent change at any of the advanced stages outlined above, i.e. plaques do not necessarily or inevitably evolve to more complex types. Furthermore, advanced lesions beyond the atheroma stage may contain regions which are characteristic of earlier or later types. Such features are usually due to focal alterations associated with plaque regression, with healing reactions following plaque disruptions or with secondary plaque formation.

C.   Plaque Neoformation

Secondary plaque formation or plaque neoformation is evidenced by foams cells infiltration and may enhance susceptibility to plaque disruption or fissuring (Figure 7a, b, c; color plate 3). Cells which connote a chronic inflammatory response are noted frequently within lesions and in the adventitia. These are usually lymphocytes and occasionally plasma ells. They may occur in clusters, often in association with apparent lytic changes in lesion matrix, suggesting an immunologically mediated development. Scattered lymphocytes are also evident in some lesions, but sections of advanced plaques may be entirely devoid of inflammatory cells. Focal lytic zones associated with such cellular infiltrates are generally small and are not likely to be detectable by ordinary imaging methods although the presence of these reactions may indicate focal plaque breakdown of potential clinical significance.

The interaction between individual and patient specific metabolic and hemodynamic risk factors are likely to determine ultimate lesion morphology and composition, the onset of hemodynamically significant stenosis as well as susceptibility to disruption. Imaging studies, particularly those which may be used to reveal differences in density and composition of plaque and wall may be used to establish plaque type providing resolution, sensitivity and specificity are sufficient to detect differences corresponding to usual plaque organization and stratification. The echogenicity of calcific deposits are likely to interfere with detailed transmedial evaluations even by intravascular ultrasound imaging.[36] It has also become evident that plaques are not of uniform composition in the axial distribution of their components. Developments of methods for examination and reconstruction of entire plaques with corresponding histopathologic validation hold the greatest promise for establishing criteria for discerning plaque type and susceptibility to disruption in the clinical setting.

V.　FEATURES INDICATIVE OF MANIFEST OR IMMINENT PLAQUE DISRUPTION

Much of our information about the composition and complication of advanced plaques is derived from the examination of highly stenotic endarterectomy specimens. Although tight stenoses correspond to large, complex plaques, it should be emphasized that images of lumen diameter on angiograms provide information regarding comparative degrees of lumen narrowing but do not provide an accurate appraisal of lesion cross-sectional area, volume or composition.[22, 32, 33] This limitation is due to the compensatory enlargement of arteries where plaques form as noted above, to changes in lumen size duet modifications of plaque modeling and composition, to the occurrence of plaque disruptions and ulcerations, to erosions of the underlying media and to the formation and organization of thrombi. Nor do focal irregularities and depressions at the lumen surface necessarily portend the presence of current ulcerations, for examination of many endarterectomy specimens and corresponding angiograms indicate that these may be regions of healing where previous thrombi or ulcerations may have occurred. Neither the degree of calcification, nor the outer vessel contour are therefore reliable indices of plaque progression, degree of stenosis or complication.

Although severe atherosclerotic disease at the carotid bifurcation frequently presents clinically as transient ischemic attacks or stroke, marked degrees of stenosis can be detected in the absence of such symptoms. Tissue vibrations created by turbulent flow distal to tight stenoses may be detected as <u>bruits</u> on physical examination and flow velocity profiles characteristic of stenoses can be detected using duplex Doppler methods.

Angiography and magnetic resonance imaging may also provide information on lumen configuration. As noted above, tight stenoses are associated with the presence of large complex plaques which tend to be complicated by ulceration, calcification, hematoma and thrombus formation even when manifest symptoms are not present clinically.[37, 38] Preemptive excision of such lesions and comparison with those removed because of retinal or cerebrovascular clinical events have permitted studies which provide insights into the nature of the morphologic changes associated with symptoms;

A. Chemical and Structural Composition of Critical Asymptomatic and Symptomatic Carotid Stenoses

Determination of the chemical composition of highly stenotic lesions have failed to reveal any significant differences between symptomatic and asymptomatic plaques (Table I). Specimens with little or only moderate stenosis and not associated with evidence of clinical symptomatology may be obtained at autopsy and compared with findings in stenotic endarterectomy specimens. In view of the axial variation in lesion composition and complication, such correlations require detailed sequential sampling. Our own studies are based on sections of the entire bifurcation taken at 0.5 cm intervals, i.e., on 6-10 sections of each specimen.[22,38,39,40] We have compared the morphologic evidences of plaque complication in endarterectomy specimens of highly stenotic plaques ($\geq$80%) with those identified in post mortem material in which stenosis was mild or moderate (<50%). For the highly stenotic endarterectomy plaques, those associated with clinical symptoms were compared with those without clinical symptoms and with the moderately stenotic plaques (Table II). One or more of the complicating features was noted in most of the specimens. Evidence of a necrotic core was present in 58% of the highly stenotic specimens and in only 12% of those with little or moderate narrowing. Ulceration was evident in 53% of the highly stenotic specimens but in only 6% of the moderately stenotic samples. Hematoma, usually within an associated necrotic core or evidence of previous hemorrhage or hematoma in the form of collections of siderophages was noted in 73% of the highly stenotic, but in only 41% of the moderately narrowed asymptomatic plaques. Calcification was a common finding, noted in 84% of the tight stenoses and 53% of the moderately narrowed arteries. These differences were significant at the $p<0.05$ to $p<0.01$ level for each finding. Thus, plaques associated with tight stenoses were more complicated than

TABLE I

SYMPTOMATIC AND ASYMPTOMATIC CAROTID ENDARTERECTOMIES WITH CRITICAL STENOSIS (>80%)			
LIPID RELATED			
	DNA (ng/mg)	**CHOLESTEROL (ug/mg**	**LIPASE (uM/mim/g)**
SYMPT (31)	182 ± 28	82 ± 18	56 ± 15
ASYMPT (14)	206 ± 50	77 ± 13	73 ± 28
CONNECTIVE TISSUE RELATED			
	COLLAGEN (ug*/mg)	**COLLAGENASE (cpm/hr/g)**	**ELASTASE (cpm/hr/g)**
SYMPT (31)	10 ± 1	190 ± 37	350 ± 50
ASYMPT (14)	11 ± 1	285 ± 84	519 ± 84

*= hydroxyproline

TABLE II

SYMPTOMATIC AND ASYMPTOMATIC CAROTID ENDARTERECTOMIES WITH CRITICAL STENOSIS (>80%)			
	HEMORRHAGE	**ULCER**	**THROMBOSIS**
SYMPT (31)	68%	58%	55%
ASYMPT (14)	85%	43%	36%
ASYMPT (1) <80% STENOSIS (AUTOPSY)	41%	6%	0%*

*+ <0.05 Compared to Symptomatic Plaque

those with moderate stenoses. When only the asymptomatic highly stenotic plaque were compared with the asymptomatic moderately stenotic post-mortem specimens, the comparisons gave similar results. Necrotic core was evident in 50% of those with tight stenosis and in 12% of those with little or moderate stenosis. Ulceration was present in 43% of the highly stenotic and only 6% of the moderately stenotic plaques. Hematoma was evidence in 86% of the tightly stenotic and 41% of the moderately stenotic. Calcification was present in 71% of the tightly stenotic and in 53% of the moderately stenotic. There were no significant differences between highly stenotic symptomatic and highly stenotic asymptomatic plaques with respect to the incidence of these complications.

These results indicate that carotid plaque complexity and predisposition to potential complications ie disruption, thrombosis, hemorrhage and embolic events is related to plaque burden and degree of luminal stenosis. In the following chapter by Badimon et al, evidence is presented which indicates that coronary plaque disruption and superimposed thrombosis may be independent of the degree of luminal stenosis occurring in soft lipid laden plaques producing moderate stenoses. This contrast between carotid and coronary plaques may be related to differences in the susceptibility of each respective vascular bed to the various atherogenic risk factors and to differences in the imposed biomechanical factors. For example, coronary plaques are subjected to cyclical bending and flexing forces by virtue of the epicardial course of the coronary arteries, while the carotid bifurcation is spared from such solid mechanical stress.

B.   Spatial Distribution of Plaque Components in Relation to the Artery Lumen

Atherosclerotic plaque disruption is considered a salient feature critical to the development of clinical ischemic manifestations in both the coronary and carotid circulation.[41,44] Although the structural features of advanced atherosclerotic plaques as well as the biomechanical forces imposed upon them have been extensively studied, the relevance of particular features of plaque morphology to fibrous cap erosion and plaque complications such as thrombosis, embolization and intraplaque has yet to be determined. As noted above carotid plaques associated with symptomatic and asymptomatic critical stenosis have similar morphologic and chemical features. Morphologic complexity appears to be related to the plaque size regardless of symptoms.[38] Conversely other investigators have observed that carotid artery plaques in symptomatic patients contained more soft cholesterol amorphous debris and hemorrhage and less collagenous material when compared to asymptomatic patients.[45,46,47] A recognized limitation inherent to the aforementioned studies is lack of precise quantitation of the individual components of the plaque and inconsistencies with regards to the selected sampling site.

As previously mentioned the presence of inflammatory cell infiltration has been associated with or proposed as a major factor in unstable, symptom producing carotid and coronary plaques.[48,50] and related to degradation of the fibrous cap and plaque neoformation. A variety of biomechanical factors have also been postulated to play a role in plaque disruption. These include mechanical stresses associated with hemodynamic wall shear or pressure fluctuations.[51-54] While advanced symptomatic and asymptomatic carotid plaques contain similar fibrous, necrotic and calcific components, we have postulated that the spatial distribution of these individual components in relation to the lumen and the extent of inflammatory cell infiltration, in particular macrophage foam cell in the abluminal fibrous cap could cannot plaque neoformation and discriminate between symptomatic and asymptomatic potential. We have examined a large number of symptomatic and asymptomatic aortic plaques with similar degrees of stenosis removed at endarterectomy.[55] In view of the relationship between plaque complexity i.e. the presence of a diversity of plaque components and plaque size or degree of stenosis; histologic sections from the most stenotic region of these plaques with respect to the relative quantity and location of the various plaque components and the proximity of these elements to each other and the lumen surface was evaluated. The degree of macrophage infiltration in and about the fibrous cap as a measure of likely plaque neoformation was also measured.

Indications for operation were symptomatic disease in 59 instances (including hemispheric TIA in 29, stroke in 19 and amaurosis fugax in 11) and angiographic asymptomatic stenosis greater than 70% in 40. Plaques removed after remote symptoms beyond 65 months were excluded. Histologic sections from the most stenotic region of the plaque were examined using computer assisted morphometry. The percent (%) area of plaque cross-section occupied by necrotic lipid core with or without associated plaque hematoma, by calcification, as well as the distance from the lumen and/or fibrous cap of each of these features, were determined. The presence of foam cells, macrophages and/or inflammatory cell collections within, upon or just beneath the fibrous cap was taken as an additional indication of plaque neoformation.

Mean % angiographic stenosis was 82 ± 11 and 79 ± 13 for the asymptomatic and symptomatic groups respectively ($p<0.05$). The necrotic core was twice as close to the lumen in symptomatic plaques when compared to asymptomatic plaques (0.27 ± 0.3 vs 0.5 ± 0.5 resp, $p<0.01$) (Figure 8) Percent area of necrotic core or calcification was similar for both groups (22% vs 26% and 7% vs 6% respectively). There was no significant relationship to symptom production of either the distance of calcification from the lumen or of the % area occupied by the lipid necrotic core or calcification.   The number of macrophages infiltrating the region of the fibrous cap was three times greater in symptomatic plaques compared to asymptomatic plaques.   Regions of fibrous cap disruption or ulceration were more commonly observed in symptomatic than in asymptomatic plaques (32% vs 20%). None of the demographic or clinical atherosclerosis risk factors distinguished between symptomatic and asymptomatic plaques.

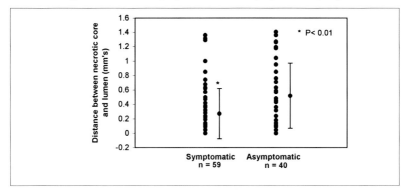

Figure 8.

It is evident from these findings that the proximity of the necrotic core to the overlying fibrous cap and lumen rather than it's absolute or percent cross-sectional area is a striking feature of symptomatic plaques. In symptomatic plaques, (Figure 9, color plate 4) the necrotic core was twice as close to the lumen when compared to asymptomatic plaques (Figure 10, color plate 5) while the degree or location of calcification had little effect. Thus, the spatial relationship among the matrix and necrotic components appear to be most important in defining likely plaque stability than content of these elements. These findings likely represent the dynamic equilibrium which exists among factors which favor fibrogenesis versus those which induce matrix degradation.[56]

Symptomatic plaques also appear to a greater degree of macrophage infiltration in and about the fibrous cap and were associated with fibrous cap thinning and erosion implicating an ongoing induction of plaque formation and or an inflammatory or immune mediated response as a factor in plaque instability. Other investigators have also noted that ruptured plaques are infiltrated by foam cells especially in regions where the fibrous cap is thinnest.[43,44,49,50,57]

Foam cells derived from mononuclear phagocytes in atherosclerotic plaques are known to elaborate a number of matrix metalloproteinases such as interstitial collagenase, gelatinase and stromelysin all of which are capable of degrading collagen, elastin and proteocoglycans.[58-61] Such processes could lead to thinning of the fibrous cap and disruption particularly if potent mechanical stresses are present. We are currently investigating the contribution of macrophage infiltration and apoptosis to the relative activity of metalloprotienases and tissue inhibitors of metalloprotienases. Preliminary results indicate that the apoptotic rate is proportional to the number of infiltrating macrophages and is related to symptomatic disease and position of the necrotic core within the plaque. Macrophage infiltration and apoptosis may modulate lesion progression and necrosis by the release of injurious free radicals and other mitogenic and tissue necrosis factors.[62-65] Activated macrophages may also induce a prothrombotic effect by inhibiting tissue plasminogen activators and thereby enhancing the thrombotic complications associated with complex atherosclerotic plaques.[66]

Interestingly plaque complications such as intraplaque hematoma and surface thrombosis, although characteristic of large advanced plaques, did not discriminate between symptomatic and asymptomatic plaques and appeared to represent events probably secondary to plaque fissuring or disruption of the fibrous cap.

The potential role of biomechanical forces in inducing structural fatigue of plaque constituents and the localization of plaque neoformation and inflammatory cell responses is under study. Marked elevation of wall shear stress occurs within a stenoses associated with large plaques. Although high shear may inhibit plaque formation[67] changes in flowdynamics associated with marked stenoses, including wall vibration, flutter, and cyclical collapse[68] could induce disruptions within plaques, lumen ulcer formation, and associated surface irregularities. Vito and others[69,70] have emphasized the relationship between plaque composition and the location of peak stress. For example, it has been found that proximity of the necrotic core to the lumen increases the stress concentration in the overlying fibrous cap. Others have demonstrated an association between regions of macrophage infiltration and mechanical stress concentration.

VI.   CONCLUSION

In summary, the specific features of carotid endarterectomy specimens which connote underlying plaque instability and correlate well with symptom production include: 1) erosion, focal narrowing or absence of the fibrous cap with or without an immediately subjacent lipid necrotic core, foam cells or an associated inflammatory cellular infiltrate, with or without demonstrable thrombus deposition, 2) the presence of hematoma within the plaque, usually in the form of blood within a necrotic core often in direct relationship to a focal surface disruption and/or the presence of clusters of siderophages, suggesting previous resolved hemorrhage or hematoma, 4) secondary lesion formation (neoformation) on an older plaque as indicated by juxtalumenal foam cell and lipid core accumulations and/or focal inflammatory cell infiltration within or upon an underlying apparently stable plaque, and 5) the juxtaposition of regions of presumably different composition and elastic modulus associated with the above-mentioned features.

Continued improvement in the resolution of existing imaging techniques with hopefully resolve such critical features of unstable carotid plaques such as fibrous cap thickness and integrity, position of necrotic core in relation to the fibrous cap and the lumen, and the relative quantity and spatial distribution of different plaque components ie. calcification, fibrous, hematoma, and necrosis. Detailed correlations between the selected imaging modality and plaque structure in the three dimensional domain will be necessary if we are to reliably utilize clinical imaging in the a) assessment of progression of regression of carotid atherosclerosis in relation to risk factors and their modification and b) detection of the unstable plaque in its predisruptive stage and prior to the development of symptoms.

References

1. Stary HC: Changes in components and structure of atherosclerotic lesions developing from childhood to middle age in coronary arteries. Basic Res Cardiol 1994; 89(Suppl I):17.
2. Stary HC, Blankenhorn DH, Chandler AB, et al: A definition of initial, fatty streak and intermediate lesions of arteriosclerosis. Circulation 1994; 89:2462.
3. Stary HC, Chandler AB, Glagov, S, et al: A definition of advanced atherosclerotic lesions and a classification of atherosclerosis. Arteriosclerosis and Thrombosis. (In press).
4. Glagov S, Zarins CK, Giddens DP: Mechanical factors in the pathogenesis, localization and evolution of atherosclerotic plaques. *In* Camilleri JP, Berry CL, Fiessinger J-N, et al (eds): Diseases of the Artery Wall. London, Springer-Verlag, 1989; pp 217.
5. Glagov S, Zarins CK, Giddens DP, et al: Establishing the hemodynamic determinants of human plaque configuration, composition and complication. *In* Yoshida Y, Yamaguchi CG, Caro S, et al (eds): Role of Blood Flow in Atherogenesis. New York, Springer-Verlag, 1988; pp 3-10.
6. Glagov S. Zarins CK, Giddens DP, et al: Hemodynamics and atherosclerosis: Insights and perspectives gained from studies of human arteries. Arch Pathol Lab Med 1988; 112:1018.
7. Taylor KE, Glagov S, Zarins CK: Preservation and structural adaptation of endothelium over experimental foam cell lesions: A quantitative ultrastructural study. Arteriosclerosis 1989; 9:881.
8. Ross R: The pathogenesis of atherosclerosis: A perspective for the 1990s. Nature 1993; 362:801.
9. Ku DN, Zarins CK, Giddens DP, et al: Pulsatile flow and atherosclerosis in the human carotid bifurcation: Positive correlation between plaque localization and low and oscillating shear stress. Arteriosclerosis 1985; 5:292.
10. Zarins CK, Giddens DP, Bjaradaj BK, et al: Carotid bifurcation atherosclerosis: Quantitative correlation of plaque localization with flow velocity profiles and wall shear stress. Circ Res 1983; 53:502.
11. Ku DN, Giddens DP: Pulsatile flow in a model carotid bifurcation. Arteriosclerosis 1983; 3:31.
12. Beere PA, Glagov S, Zarins CK: Experimental atherosclerosis at the carotid bifurcation of the cynomolgus monkey: Localization, compensatory enlargement and the sparing effect of heart rate. Arteriosclerosis and Thrombosis 1992; 12:1245.
13. Beere PA, Glagov S, Zarins CK: Retarding effect of lowered heart rate on coronary atherosclerosis. Science 1984; 226:180.
14. Clark JM, Glagov S: Transmural organization of the arterial wall: the lamellar unit revisited. Arteriosclerosis 1985; 5:19-34.
15. Kamiya A, Togawa T: Adaptive regulation of wall shear stress to flow change in the canine aortic artery. Am J Physiol 1990l; 239:H14-H21.
16. Zarins CK, Zatina MA, Giddens DP, Ku DN, Glagov S: Shear stress regulation of artery lumen diameter in experimental atherogenesis. J Vasc Surg 1987; 5:413-420.
17. Wolinsky H, Glagov S: A lamellar unit of aortic medial structure and function in mammals. Circulation Res. 1967; 20:99-111.
18. Leung DYM, Glagov S, Mathews MB: Elastin and collagen accumulation in rabbit ascending aorta and pulmonary trunk during postnatal growth: correlation of cellular synthetic response with medial tension. Circulation Res 1977; 41:316-323.
19. Bassiouny HS, Lieber BB, Giddens DP, Xu CP, Glagov S, Zarins CZ: Quantitative inverse correlation of wall shear stress with experimental intimal thickening. Surgical Forum 1988; 39:328-30.
20. Zarins, CK, Giddens DP, Bharadvaj BK, Sottiuurai VS, Mabon RF, Glagov S. Carotid bifurcation atherosclerosis: quantitative correlation of plaque localization with flow velocity profiles and wall shear stress. Circ Res 1983; 53:502-514.
21. Masawa N, Glagov S, Zarins CK: Quantitative morphologic study of intimal thickening at the human carotid bifurcation. I. Axial and circumferential distribution of maximum intimal thickening in asymptomatic uncomplicated plaques. Atherosclerosis 1994; 107:137-146.
22. Masawa N, Glagov S, Zarins CK: Quantitative morphologic study of intimal thickening at the human carotid bifurcation. II. The compensatory enlargement response and the role of the intima in tensile support. Atherosclerosis 1994; 107:147-155.
23. Ku DN, Zarins CK, Giddens DP, Glagov S: Pulsatile flow and atherosclerosis in the human carotid bifurcation: positive correlation between plaque localization and low and oscillating shear stress. Arteriosclerosis 1985; 5:292-303.
24. Caro CG, Fitz-Gerald JM, Schroter BC: Arterial wall shear and distribution of early atheroma in man. Nature 1969; 223:1159-1161.
25. Svindland A: The localization of sudanophilic and fibrous plaques in the main left coronary arteries. Atherosclerosis 1983; 48:139-145.
26. Thubrikar MJ, Baker JW, Nolan SP: Inhibition of atherosclerosis associated with reduction of arterial intramural stress in rabbits. Arteriosclerosis 1988; 8:410-420, 1988.

27. Tracy RE, Kissling GE, Curtis MB: Smooth muscle cell-reticulin lamellar units of 13.2 μm thickness composing the aortic intima. Virchows Arch A 1987; 411:415-424.
28. Stary HC, Chandler AB, Glagov S, Guyton JR, Insull W Jr., Rosenfield ME, et al.: A definition of intimal, fatty streak and intermediate lesions of arteriosclerosis. Circulation 1994; 89:2462-2478.
29. Stary HC, Chandler AB, Dinsmore RE, et al: A definition of advanced type of atherosclerotic lesions and a histological classification of atherosclerosis. Arteriosclerosis and Thrombosis: (In press).
30. Ku DN, Giddens DP: Pulsatile flow in a model carotid bifurcation. Arteriosclerosis 1983; 3:31-39.
31. Frank JS, Fogelman AM: Ultrastructure of the intimal in WHHL and cholesterol-fed rabbit aortas prepared by ultra-rapid freezing and freeze-etching. J Lipid Res 1989; 30:967-978.
32. Glagov S, Weisenberg E, Zarins CK, Stankunavicius R, Kolettis G: Compensatory enlargement of human atherosclerotic coronary arteries. N Engl J Med 1987; 316:1371-1375.
33. Zarins CK, Weisenberg E, Kolettis G, Stankunavicius R, Glagov S: Differential enlargement of artery segments in response to enlarging atherosclerosis plaques. J Vas Surg 1988; 7:386-394.
34. Ko C, Glagov S, Zarins CK: Structural basis for the compensatory enlargement of arteries during early atherogenesis. Proceedings of the 3rd International Workshop on Vascular Hemodynamics (Bologna, 1991) Gorgatti E, ed. Centro Scientifico Editore 1992; pp 157-161.
35. Evans CH, Georgescu HI, Lin CW, Mendelow D, Steed DL, Webster MW: Inducible synthesis of collagenase by cells of aortic origin. J Surg Res 1991; 42:328-330.
36. Keren G, Leon MB: Intravascular ultrasound of atherosclerotic vessels: changes observed during interventional procedures. Am J Cardiac Imaging 1994; 8:129-139.
37. Hatsukami TS, Thackray BD, Primozich JF, et al. Echolucent regions in carotid plaque: prelaminar analysis comparing three-dimensional histologic reconstructions to sonographic findings. Ultrasound in Medicine & Biology 1994; 20(8):743-749.
38. Bassiouny HS, Davis H, Masawa N, et al. Critical carotid stenosis: morphological and chemical similarity between symptomatic and asymptomatic plaques. J Vasc Surg 1989; 9:202-212.
39. Masawa N, Glagov S, Zarins CK. Quantitative morphologic study of intimal thickening at the human carotic bifurcation. I. Axial and circumferential distribution of maximum intimal thickening in asymptomatic uncomplicated plaques. Atherosclerosis 1994; 107:137-146.
40. Glagov S, Masawa N, Bassiouny H, et al. Morphologic bases for establishing end-points for early plaque detection and plaque stability. International J Cardiac Imaging, 1995; 4:1-7.
41. Carr SA, Farb A, Pearce WH, et al. Atherosclerotic plaque rupture in symptomatic carotid artery stenosis. (In press).
42. Fuster V, Stein B, Ambrose JA, et al. Atherosclerotic plaque rupture and thrombosis: Evolving concepts. Circulation 1990; 82:(SII):47-59.
43. Falk E. Why do plaques rupture? Circulation 1992; 86:(SIII):30-42.
44. Falk E, Shah PK, Fuster V. Coronary plaque disruption. Circulation 1995; 92:657-671.
45. Feely TM, Leen EJ, Colgan MP, et al. Histologic characteristics of the carotid artery plaque. J Vasc Surg 1991; 3:719-724.
46. Seeger JM, Klingman N. The relationship between carotid plaque composition and neurologic symptoms. J Surg Res 1987; 43:78-85.
47. Geroulakos G, Ramaswami G, Nicolaides A, et al. Characterization of symptomatic and asymptomatic carotid plaques using high-resolution real-time ultrasonography. Br J Surgery, 80(10):1274-1277, 1993.
48. Hansson GK, Jonasson L, Seifert PS, et al. Immune mechanisms in atherosclerosis. Arteriosclerosis 1989; 9:567-578.
49. Mazzone A, De Servi S, Ricevuti G, et al. Increased expression of neutrophil and monocyte adhesion molecules in unstable coronary artery disease. Circulation 1993; 88:358-363.
50. Moreno PR, Falk E, Palacios IF, et al. Macrophage infiltration in acute coronary syndromes: Implications for plaque rupture. Circulation 1994; 90:775-778, 1994.
51. Gertz SD, Robert WC. Hemodynamic shear forces in rupture of coronary arterial atherosclerotic plaque. Am J Cardiol 1990; 66:1368-1372.
52. Loree HM, Kamm RD, Atkinson CM, et al. Turbulent pressure fluctuation on surface of model vascular stenosis. Am J Physiol 1991; 261:H664-H650.
53. Binns RL, Ku DN. Effect of stenosis on wall motion; A possible mechanisms of stroke and transient ischemic attack. Arteriosclerosis 1989; 261:H644-H650.
54. Muller JE, Rofler GH, Stone PH. Circadian variation and triggers of onset of acute cardiovascular disease. Circulation 1989; 79:733-743.
55. Bassiouny HS, Sakaguchi Y, Mikucki SA, McKinsey JF, Piano G, Gewertz BL, and Glagov S. Juxtalumenal location of plaque necrosis and neoformation in symptomatic carotid stenosis. J Vasc Surg. (In press.).
56. Hennerici M, Trockel U, Rautenberg W, et al. Spontaneous progression and regression of small carotid atheroma. Lancet 1985; pp 1415-1419.

57. Lendon CL, Davies MJ, Born GVR, et al. Atherosclerotic plaques are locally weakened when macrophage density is increased. Atherosclerosis 1991; 87:87-90.

58. Welgus HG, Campbell EJ, Cury JD, et al. Differential susceptibility of type X collagen to cleavage by two mammalian interstitial collagenases and 72-KD a type IV collagenase. J Biol Chem 1990; 265:13521-13527.

59. Chin JR, Murphy G, Werb Z. Stromelysin, a connective tissue degrading metal loendopeptidase secreted by stimulated rabbit synovial fibroblasts in parallel with collagenase. J Biol Chem 1985; 260:12367-12376.

60. Henney AM, Wakekey PR, David MJ, et al. Location of stromelysin gene in atherosclerotic plaques using in situ hybridization. PNAS USA 1991; 88:8154-8158.

61. Brown DL, Hibbs MS, Kearney M, et al. Expression and cellular location of 92 Kda gelatinase in coronary lesions of patients with unstable angina. J AM Coll Cardiol Special issue 1994; 123A. Abstract.

62. Galis ZS, Sukhova GK, Lark MW, et al. Increased expression of matrix metalloproteinases and matrix degrading activity in vulnerable regions of human atherosclerotic plaques. J Clin Invest 1994; 94:2493-2503,

63. Tipping PG, Hancock WW. Production of tumor necrosis factor and interleukin-1 by macrophages from human atheromatous plaques. Am J Pathol 1993; 142:1721-1728.

64. Clinton SK, Underwood R, Hayes L, et al. Macrophage colony-stimulating factor gene expression in vascular cells and in experimental and human atherosclerosis. Am J Pathol 1992;. 140:301-306.

65. Geng Y, Libby P. Evidence for apoptosis in advanced human atheroma; colocalization with interleukin-b β-converting enzyme. Am J Pathol 147:251-226, 1995.

66. Emeis JJ, Kooistra T. Interleukin and lipopolysaccharide induce an inhibitor of tissue-type plasminogen activator in vivo and in cultured endothelial cells. J Exp Med 163-:1260-1266, 1986.

67. Zarins CK, Bomberger RA, Glagov S. Local effects of stenoses; increased flow velocity inhibits atherogenesis. Circulation 64:221-227, 1981.

68. Cancelli C, Pedley TJ. A separated flow model for collapsible rube oscillations. J Fluid Mech 157:375-404, 1985.

69. Vito RP, Whang MC, Giddens DP, et al. Stress analysis of the diseased arterial cross-section, ASME Adv Bioeng Proc pp 273-276, 1990.

70. Richardson PD, Davies MJ, Born GVR. Influence of plaque configuration and stress distribution and fissuring of coronary atherosclerotic plaque. Lancet 2:941-944, 1989.

THE ROLE OF ATHEROSCLEROTIC PLAQUE DISRUPTION AND THROMBOSIS IN ACUTE CORONARY HEART DISEASE

*Juan J. Badimon, Ph.D. , Richard Gallo, M.D., Lina Badimon, Ph.D.,
James H. Chesebro, M.D. and Valentin Fuster, M.D., Ph.D.*

*Cardiovascular Biology Research Laboratory
Cardiovascular Institute
Mount Sinai School of Medicine
New York, New York U.S.A.*

Contents

I. INTRODUCTION

Atherosclerosis is a focal pathological phenomena characterized by arterial thickening and hardening. Recently, epidemiological and experimental studies have identified several risk factors that are relevant in patients with atherosclerotic disease. Among them, hyperlipidemia appears to plays a major role in atherogenesis while thrombotic complications are thought to be the major trigger of acute events in the coronary circulation. In this review, we will briefly discuss the pathogenesis of atherosclerosis and the morphological characteristics of arterial lesions with emphasis on the role of thrombosis in plaque progression.

II. HYPOTHESIS ON THE ORIGIN OF ATHEROSCLEROSIS

The two major factors are thought to be at the origin of atherosclerosis, the thrombotic and lipidic. Thrombus as an etiologic factor for atherosclerosis first described by von Rokitansky (1), and suggests that fibrin organization by fibroblasts, associated with further lipid enrichment, would lead to intimal thickening. This theory has been supported by the observation of fibrin-, and platelet-rich thrombi in atherosclerotic plaques. In addition more recently, platelet activation has been shown as an important mediator of vascular smooth muscle cell migration and proliferation (2,3).

Accumulation of lipid within the arterial wall is the consequence of an increased deposition of plasma lipids in the wall and is related to imbalance between the mechanisms responsible for the ingress and removal of lipids (4). The possibility of inducing atherosclerotic-like lesions in several animal species and the direct relationship between high plasma levels of lipids and incidence of atherosclerotic disease in humans, clearly support this hypothesis.

These two initiating factors can be combined into a single multifactorial theory that involves one common step, endothelial dysfunction, which triggers the successive events responsible for the formation of atherosclerotic lesions (5-7) (See Table 1). The coexistence of one or more of the risk factors (elevated LDL-cholesterol, smoking, diabetes, high blood pressure and low HDL-cholesterol levels) and their direct and indirect local hemorheological effects could contribute to the induction of an endothelial lesion. A break in the endothelial barrier will facilitate the entrance of circulating monocytes and plasma lipids into the arterial wall, as well as platelet deposition at the sites of endothelial denudation. Damaged endothelial cells, monocytes, and aggregated platelets through the release of mitogenic factors, such as platelet derived growth factor (PDGF), potentiates the migration and proliferation of vascular SMC; together with increased receptor-mediated lipid accumulation and increased connective tissue synthesis, would shape the typical atheromatous plaque. Perpetuation of these processes may account for the slow progression of the disease. However, in some instances a much faster development is observed; thrombosis associated with a disrupted or ruptured plaque seems to be responsible for this process.

Table 1.   *Multifactorial origin of atherosclerosis*

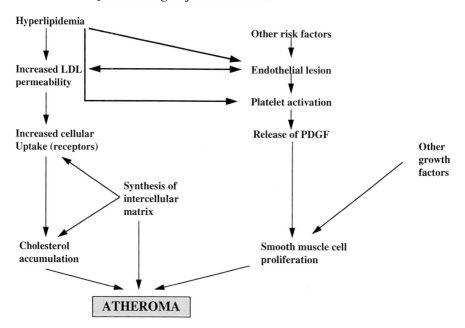

II. EVOLUTION OF ATHEROSCLEROTIC LESIONS

Atherosclerotic disease affects mainly the medium and large-sized arteries, such as the aorta, carotid, cerebral, and renal. Recently, HC Stary (8) provided a comprehensive description of atherosclerotic plaque morphology. The different histopathologic types or stages of the disease have been described in the preceding chapter and are represented in Figure I. The cellular and molecular mechanisms underlying the induction and progression of atherosclerosis are summarized in the subsequent section.

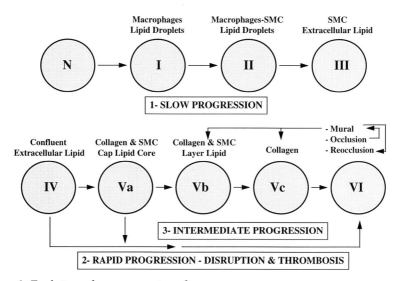

Figure 1. Evolution of coronary artery disease

A.   The Early Lesion (Stary type I, II)

Atherosclerotic lesions tend to develop in lesion prone areas, as in arterial bifurcations, which are subject to repeated mechanical forces, such as oscillating shear forces (9-10). The endothelium at these sites is dysfunctional and characterized by increased permeability leading to an influx of low-density lipoproteins (LDL) and other plasma proteins into the intima (11-12).

Additionally, circulating monocytes adhere to activated endothelial cells (expressing adhesive cell-surface glycoproteins such as E-selectin, VCAM-1 or ICAM-1)(13-14), migrate between endothelial cells, where they enter the intima and differentiate into macrophages which can endocytose native and oxidized LDL. Lipids can also accumulate indirectly after death of lipid-rich foam cells (15).

Recent pathologic evidence suggests that the lipid rich core originates primarily from lipoprotein trapping and binding to matrix proteins such as glycosaminoglycans, collagen and fibrinogen (16-18), this process results in focal collections of lipid laden foam cells seen microscopically as yellow fatty clots or streaks raised above the intimal surface (Stary type II).

B.   Mature Plaques (Stary Type III, IV)

The initial lipid and macrophage driven process is subsequently accompanied by smooth muscle cell activation, migration, and proliferation, followed by extracellular matrix deposition and further lipid accumulation. This gives rise to the more mature and clinically significant atherosclerotic plaques (Stary type III, VI, V) (19-20). The endothelium is intact but dysfunctional in the early phases of atherosclerosis. Later the endothelium is often physically and functionally impaired by the further recruitment of monocytes and macrophages (21-22), compounded by the toxic effects of oxidized LDL, and degradation products such as oxygen free-radicals (15). Platelets and thrombi are often found adherent to areas of endothelial denudation, and can become incorporated into the atherosclerotic plaque (5-7). Furthermore platelet derived growth factors and thrombin, generated by the intrinsic and extrinsic coagulating pathways, have been found to possess chemotactic and mitogenic properties (23) that can contribute to plaque growth by stimulating adjacent smooth muscle cells.

C. The Vulnerable Plaques (Stary Type IV and V)

Atherosclerosis is a multifocal disease. The coronary arteries are generally diffusely involved with confluent plaques carpeting the vessel wall (24), but individual plaques vary greatly in composition. In patients presenting with acute coronary syndromes, a significant atheromatous core is present in the majority of unstable plaques (25).

Fibrous plaques (Stary types VII) are stable and often resistant to disruption, but may produce stable angina if coronary blood flow is reduced (Figure 2, color plate 5).

A vulnerable fibrolipid plaque consists of a lipid-rich core separated from the arterial lumen by a fibromuscular cap. This atheromatous core is mostly avascular (26-27), hypocellular (except at the periphery where macrophage foam cells are frequently present), devoid of supporting collagen, rich in free cholesterol esters and very soft (28-29) (Figure

(Figure 2, Color Plate 5). In postmortem studies the atheromatous gruel has a toothpaste-like consistency at room temperature and is even softer at body temperature in vivo. Not surprisingly, soft plaques are less stable and more vulnerable to rupture. Plaque rupture frequently occurs where the fibrous cap is thinnest, and most heavily infiltrated with foam cells and macrophages. This region of the plaque is also subjected to peak stress loading as all physical forces acting here are greatest. For eccentric plaques description is observed in the shoulder region at the junction of the plaque with the less diseased adjacent vessel wall (30-32).

The atheromatous gruel, is considered highly thrombogenic(32). With plaque disruption, exposure of the contents of the necrotic core to the flowing blood may result in thrombus formation and subsequent lumen narrowing or occlusion. Recent studies suggest that the high thrombogenicity of disrupted atherosclerotic plaques is mediated by tissue factor (34-37). Therefore, nonstenotic but soft plaques should be considered ominous since myocardial infarction may often result from acute occlusion related to disrupted lipid-laden lesions. These observations suggest limiting the management of coronary artery disease to severely stenotic atherosclerotic plaques may not entirely prevent sudden myocardial infarction.

IV. ATHEROSCLEROTIC PLAQUE PROGRESSION

The progression of early atherosclerotic lesions to the most developed, clinically evident lesions, is often more rapid in those subjects with the coexistence of more than one risk factors, and in lesions with certain morphologic characteristics (38). Some plaques experience a slow progression, probably as a consequence of the complex biological sequence of events previously discussed. However, there is also a faster and more clinically significant explosive growth affecting the most fatty or cell-rich atherosclerotic plaques, characterized by the presence of an acute thrombotic event and its subsequent fibrotic organization.

A. Slow Plaque Progression

Based on pathological evidence, the slow progression of some atherosclerotic plaques would be the consequence of the following biochemical events (Table I). The existence of an endothelial dysfunction (Type I lesion) facilitates the internalization of circulating lipids and monocytes. The perpetuation of these processes is associated with the formation of foam cells, release of mitogenic and growth factors, along with increased synthesis of connective tissue by the proliferating SMC. High levels of cell cholesterol would induce the death of these lipid-laden cells with the release of their lipid content and formation of an extracellular lipid core. Usually these plaques are characterized by a clinically silent progression, since their slow and temporally linear growth rate may permit the development of collaterals that support the distal demand for blood.

B. Rapid Plaque Progression.

Acute thrombus formation on a disrupted atherosclerotic plaque is fundamental in the onset of acute ischemic events, has been demonstrated in autopsy studies of patients who expire suddenly or shortly after a coronary event (25, 29, 38-41). Emerging evidence suggests that plaque rupture, subsequent thrombosis, and fibrous organization of thrombus are important in the progression of atherosclerosis in asymptomatic patients and those with stable angina. In addition, within the past few years it has become apparent that coronary atherosclerotic lesions with less severe angiographic disease are associated with rapid progression to severe stenosis or total occlusion and that these lesions may account for up to two-thirds of patients in whom unstable angina or acute myocardial infarction develops (42-43). Post-mortem angiographic studies have shown that eccentric lesions with irregular borders commonly represent plaque rupture, hemorrhage, partially occluding or recanalized thrombi (44-45). Studies on atherosclerotic plaques have revealed old, organized thrombi that were difficult to differentiate from atherosclerotic changes seen in the arterial wall. According to these observations, organization of thrombi contributes to the progression to advanced atherosclerotic plaques. A detailed study in patients with unstable angina leading to infarction or sudden death revealed thrombi with a layered appearance in most cases (46). These observations suggest that several consecutive mild episodes of mural thrombosis may occur and eventually lead to critical vascular occlusion. Thus, plaque disruption with mural thrombus formation and its subsequent fibrotic organization may be potential mechanism in the fast progression of atherosclerotic plaques.

V.   PLAQUE COMPOSITION AND INSTABILITY

Rupture of the fibrous cap overlying the atheromatous core exposes thrombogenic material to the blood plasma. A mass of platelet right thrombus forms on site of disruption leading to plaque expansion. Ultimately the intraluminal thrombus may grow to become totally occlusive or progressive lysed. The plaque fissure reseals and becomes incorporated within the atheromatous plaque. Over the site of rupture luminal thrombi are not necessarily occlusive, in fact in hours or days lumen is reshaped and flow restored to different degrees (38).

Plaque tears run more often longitudinally than transversely, most are microscopic but when intraintimal thrombosis or luminal thrombosis is significant the tear may be visible on gross examination (31).

Plaque disruption is a clinically relevant phenomenon. In early work by Constantinides, thrombi causing myocardial infarction, (reconstructed from serial sections of coronary arteries) would be traced to cracks or fissures into a plaque (47). Further work by other investigators have convincingly shown that plaque rupture underlies the majority of anatomic events responsible for acute coronary syndromes (25, 38-41).

This risk of plaque disruption is essentially a function of two variables. One of them is intrinsic to the specific pathoanatomic features of the plaque, such as the relative content of fibrotic or lipid composition and amount of cellular elements present such as percentage of macrophages versus smooth muscle cell populating the atherosclerotic plaque. the second is a sum of all external physical, hemodynamic and pathophysiological forces acting on plaques, which can precipitate plaque rupture.

VI.   PLAQUE COMPOSITION AND THROMBOGENICITY

Platelet-vessel wall interaction and thrombus formation is modulated by the interaction of local rheology, the nature of the exposed substrate and systemic factors.

Local rheology is a function of the severity of the residual stenosis after plaque disruption and surface irregularities on the residual plaque. The higher the degree of stenosis and the roughness of the substrate are associated with a larger platelet-thrombus formation (33) as a consequence of the increased local shear rate conditions.

The nature of the exposed substrate is related to the severity and extent of disruption as well as the composition of the exposed substrate to flowing blood. As shown in figure

2, there is a marked heterogeneity in the composition of human atherosclerotic plaques that could be found in the same individual. Therefore, disruption of different plaques exposes different vessel wall components to blood. Data on the thrombogenicity of disrupted atherosclerotic lesions is limited. Our group has studied the relative thrombogenicity of atherosclerotic plaque components. Different human atherosclerotic plaques were exposed to flowing blood and their thrombogenicity evaluated. The studied aortic plaques were classified as normal intima (disease-free), fatty streaks, sclerotic plaques, fibrolipid plaques and atheromatous lipid rich core. From all the substrates, the atheromatous plaque, characterized by the presence of a lipid core abundant in cholesterol crystals, displayed the highest thrombogenicity (Figure 3, color plate 6).

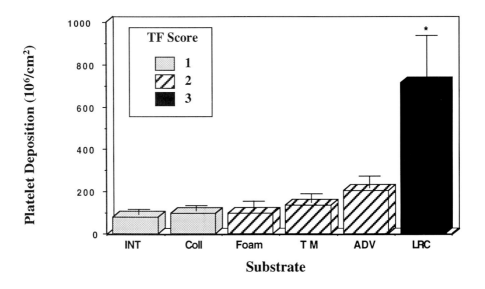

Figure 4. Platelet disposition and Tissue Factor Activity Score. INT: normal intima, Coll: collagen-rich matrix, Foam: foam cell-rich matrix, TM: normal tunica media, ADV: adventitia and LRC: lipid-rich core. (*p=0.0002.) (from ref. 40).

Tissue factor antigen and activity have been reported in human atherosclerotic plaques (34-37), we have recently reported a positive correlation (Figure 4) between human plaque thrombogenicity and their tissue factor content (37). This observation suggest that tissue factor is an important determinant of thrombogenicity after spontaneous or mechanical human atherosclerotic plaque disruption. Therefore, new therapeutic approaches specifically directed towards the tissue factor pathway of coagulation may offer promising new tools for preventing thrombotic occlusion in patients with unstable angina, or reocclusion after successful thrombolysis, or percutaneous coronary angioplasty.

Among the systemic factors that have been associated with an increased incidence of thrombotic coronary events are platelet hyperaggregability, a hypercoagulable state, and impaired fibrinolysis (7).

VII. ARTERIAL THROMBOSIS: THE CLINICAL MANIFESTATIONS OF ATHEROSCLEROSIS

The clinical manifestations of atherosclerotic plaques depend on several factors including; the degree and suddenness of blood flow obstruction, the duration of decreased myocardial perfusion and the myocardial oxygen demand at the time of blood flow obstruction. The thrombotic response to the disrupted plaque is also a major determinant. Plaque rupture is accompanied by hemorrhage into the plaque and is accompanied by various amounts of luminal thrombosis. If the thrombus is small, plaque rupture will likely be a clinically silent event. If on the other hand the thrombus is large, compromising blood flow to the myocardium the individual may experience an acute ischemic syndrome.

The incidence of thrombi in unstable angina varied significantly among different studies, in part related to the time interval between anginal symptoms and arteriographic study. The shorter this interval the higher the likelihood of finding occlusive thrombi.

It is likely that when injury to the vessel wall is mild, the thrombogenic stimulus is relatively limited and the resulting thrombotic occlusion transient, as occurs in unstable angina. On the other hand, deep vessel injury secondary to plaque rupture and ulceration results in exposure of collagen, lipids and other elements of the arterial media, leading to relatively persistent thrombotic occlusion and myocardial infarction.

It should be noted that mechanisms other than plaque fissuring and thrombosis may underly coronary events. Hemodynamic, electrocardiographic and angiographic monitoring suggest that coronary vasospasm also plays an important role in the pathogenesis of ischemic heart diseases. In unstable angina, release of vasoactive substances by both platelet and arterial wall, may contribute to a reduction of coronary blood flow. Vasospasm was found to be an important contributor to intermittent coronary occlusion in patients with acute myocardial infarction treated with intracoronary streptokinase, which respond, in some cases, to the administration of nitrates.

VIII. PREVENTION OF PLAQUE DISRUPTION

A plaque's intrinsic vulnerability and extrinsic rupture triggers are the two key determinants for plaque rupture and represent the principle targets for prevention of coronary vascular events.

A. Plaque Stabilization

Human atherosclerotic plaques can be stabilized against disruption by antiatherogenic therapy, including modifications of lifestyle and serum lipids (48-52). Numerous lipid-lowering trials with angiographic follow-up have independently demonstrated that significant clinical benefits (reduction in the incidence of myocardial infarction, unstable angina, and death) are associated with minimal regression in coronary plaque burden (48-55). For example the Familial Atherosclerosis Treatment Study (FATS trial) produced only a 1% mean regression of coronary stenoses with lipid-lowering agents. However, this translated into a striking 73% reduction in cardiovascular events. This and other similar results may signal an effect of therapies on plaque composition and stability. Collectively these trials did not demonstrate significant regression, but they did show a slowing of the progression of atherosclerotic lesions. One could speculate that this is because of a reduced incidence of plaque growth (cyclic plaque rupture and thrombosis).

The atheromatous core of most vulnerable plaques are rich in soft, semi-liquid - cholesterol esters. Theoretically, by reducing the liquid cholesterol ester content and increasing the relative content of the remaining harder crystalline cholesterol, and fibrous tissue, lipid-lowering therapy may result in stiffer, more stable lesions. Additionally, reduction in the level of circulating LDL-cholesterol, reduces the amount of cholesterol entering the plaque, and permits increased cholesterol clearance from the plaque by HDL (56).

Recent large clinical trials showing a direct beneficial effect of lipid-lowering drugs on the reduction of clinical events, suggest that the observed clinical benefits are a consequence of the stabilization of atherosclerotic plaques. The Scandinavian Simvastatin Survival Study (57), the West of Scotland Coronary Prevention Study (58), and the Cholesterol and Recurrent Events (CARE) group of investigators (59) have demonstrated that the incidence of coronary heart disease could be dramatically reduced by lowering lipid levels in a population with or without clinically manifest coronary disease. Similar results have been confirmed in a metaanalysis of four smaller regression trials using pravastatin as a lipid lowering drug (60).

Other approaches that may reduce the incidence of plaque rupture include angiotensin-converting enzyme (ACE) inhibitors. ACE-inhibitors influence both plaque vulnerability and triggering mechanisms responsible for disease onset. ACE activity may contribute to the development of coronary artery disease (61). Results from the large SAVE (62-64) and SOLVD (65-66) trials point to a reduction of 14% to 28% in the incidence of myocardial infarction and other ischemic events in patients with left ventricular dysfunction. The mechanisms for this reduction are uncertain. Angiotensin II is a growth factor for smooth muscle cells and ACE-inhibitors can reduce intimal hyperplasia after endothelial injury (67). However, it is unclear whether these agents modulate strictly atherogenesis.

Oxidized LDL is a powerful activator of macrophages, and is toxic for surrounding tissue. A plaque's content in oxidized LDL, and macrophages can be theoretically reduced with the use of antioxidants (68-69). Initial experiments in animal model of atherosclerosis showed promising reduction in atherosclerosis with the powerful antioxidant, probucol. However, the recent Probucol Quantitative Regression Swedish Trial (PQRST) failed to show a reduction in femoral artery atherosclerosis using the same agent (70).

The role of dietary antioxidant vitamins in preventing coronary heart disease and cancer has aroused considerable interest since it was reported that these vitamins interfere passively with the oxidative damage to DNA and lipoproteins (71-72). Recently a large epidemiologic study failed to demonstrate any beneficial effect of more than 12 years of beta-carotene supplementation on the incidence of malignant neoplasm (73). Similar data were reported in another trial after 4 years of beta-carotene and vitamin A supplementation

(74). On the other hand, Kushi et al reported that the intake of vitamin E-containing food is inversely associated with the risk of death from coronary heart disease in postmenopausal women (75). The Cambridge Heart Antioxidant Study (CHAOS) study suggested a reduction in the incidence of non-fatal myocardial infarction with larger doses of supplements (76). It has been shown that generous intake of vegetable, fruits and grains lower the risk of death from cardiovascular diseases and cancer. Therefore, antioxidants may not account for all the benefits associated with this dietary pattern (77). Large epidemiological trials have reported up to a 50% reduction in the rate of cardiovascular mortality in postmenopausal women treated with estrogen replacement therapy (78). Estrogens can increase a women's HDL cholesterol level, and lower LDL cholesterol levels. They also have direct anti-ischemic effects such as coronary artery vasodilation. Recently, an enhanced fibrinolytic activity among women undergoing hormone replacement therapy has been reported (79). However, the effect of estrogens on coronary artery disease progression is under investigation and remains to be determined.

B.   Trigger Reduction

Of all secondary risk factors, smoking is the most important preventable cause of morbidity and mortality from coronary artery disease (80). Smoking accelerates coronary artery disease (81-82), but fortunately this increased risk is rapidly reversible by cessation (83). Smoking appears to impair endothelial function, and promote lipid oxidation. Furthermore smoking is related to increases in catecholamine release, enhanced platelet aggregability, and thrombin generation.

ß-blockers may reduce the incidence of plaque rupture. The lower the heart rate the better the protection against reinfarction and sudden death (84). ß-blockers reduce circumferential wall tension (by reduction in blood pressure, and blunting of catecholamine surges), and both radial and axial stresses (by reduction in pulse pressure). By reducing the frequency and force of cyclic bending and stretching, ß-blockers may reduce cap fatigue.

The renin-angiotensin system can interfere with endogenous fibrinolysis. Patients with high renin hypertension are at higher risk of myocardial infarction then patients with low-renin hypertension. ACE-inhibitors may indirectly enhance endogenous fibrinolysis, resulting in a reduced thrombotic response to plaque rupture (85). A review of evidence from clinical trials has recently been reported (86).

In conclusion, future progress in the prevention and management of coronary ischemic events will be prediated on the early and precise identification of the vulverable athersclerotic plaque. Current evidence would suggest that plaque disruption and superimposed thrombosis in the coronary tree may occur not only in severe flow limiting stenoses but also in moderate nonhemodynamically significant plaques. Thus, the structural composition of the coronary plaque plays a critical role in determining clinical outcome. Early identification of the vulnerable plaques prior to disruption remains a challenging goal. Recent advances in high resolution imaging techniques such as intravascular ultrasound may potentially provide insight into the in vivo architecture of the plaque with regards to integrity of the fibrous cap, and the distribution of necrotic, fibrous and calcific plaque components.

Correlation of these findings with clinical outcome and in relation to corresponding histopathologic features and individual patient risk profile will help in better prospective assessment of interventions designed to regress and stabilize plaques prone to disruption and thrombosis.

References

1.   Von Rokitansky C: A manual of pathological anatomy. Vol. 4 Berlin, Syndheman Soc 1852. p 261.
2.   Ross R:The pathogenesis of atherosclerosis an update. N Engl J Med 1986; 314:488.
3.   Bini A, Fenoglio J, Mesa-Tejada et al. Identification and distribution of fibrinogen, fibrin and degradation products in atherosclerosis. Arteriosclerosis 1989; 9:109-121.
4.   Anitschkow N, Chalatow S: Uber experimentelle cholesterinstectase and ibre Bedentung fur die Entstehung einiger pathologischer Prozsse Centralbl Allg Path v Path Anot 24, 1:1913.
5.   Badimon JJ, Fuster V, Chesebro J, Badimon L. Coronary Atherosclerosis. A Multifactorial Disease. Circulation 1993; 87:(Suppl II) 3-16.
6.   Fuster V, Badimon L, Badimon JJ, Chesebro JH. The pathogenesis of coronary artery disease and the acute coronary syndromes. N Engl J Med. Parts 1 and 2, 1992; 326: 242-250 and 310-318.
7.   Fuster V. Lewis A. Conner Memorial Lecture: Mechanisms leading to myocardial infarction: insights from studies of vascular biology. Circulation. 1994; 90:2126-46.
8.   Stary HC: Composition and classification of human atherosclerotic lesions. Virchows Archiv A Pathol Anat 1992; 421:277-290.
9.   Glagov Z, Zarins CK, Giddens DP, Ku DN. Hemodynamics and atherosclerosis. Insights and perspectives gained from studies of human arteries. Arch Pathol Lab Med 1988; 112:1018-1031.
10.   Stary HC, Blankenhorn DH, Chandler AB, Glagov S, Insull W, Richardson M, et al. A definition of the intima of human arteries and of its atherosclerosis-prone regions. A report from the committee on vascular lesions of the council on Atherosclerosis, American Heart Association. Circulation 1992; 85:391-405.
11.   Ross R. The pathogenesis of atherosclerosis: A perspective for the 1990s. Nature 1993; 362:801-809.
12.   Johnson-Tidey RR, McGregor JL, Taylor PR, Poston RN. Increase in adhesion molecule P-selectin in endothelium overlying atherosclerotic plaques. Am J Pathol 1994; 144:952-961.
13.   Rosenfeld ME, Pestel E. Cellularity of atherosclerotic lesions. Coron Art Dis. 1994; 5:189-197.
14.   Navab M, Hama SY, Nguyen TB, Fogelman AM. Monocyte adhesion and transmigration in atherosclerosis. Coron Art Dis 1994; 5:198-204.
15.   Guyton JR, Klemp KF. Development of the lipid-rich core in human atheroscerlosis. Thromb Vasc Biol. 1996; 16:4-11.
16.   Guyton JR, Klemp KF. Transitional features in human atherosclerosis. Intimal thickening, cholesterol clefts, and cell loss in human aortic fatty streaks. Am J Pathol 1993; 143:1444-1457.
17.   Guyton JR, Klemp KF. Development of atherosclerotic core region. Chemical and ultrastructural analysis of microdiseased atherosclerotic lesions from human aorta. Arterioscler Thromb 1994; 14:1305-1314.
18.   Berenson GS, Radhakrishnamurthy B, Srinivasan R, Vijayagopal P, Dalferes ER. Arterial wall injury and proteoglycan changes in atherosclerosis. Atherosclerosis 1998; 112:1002-1010.
19.   Schwartc CJ, Valente AJ, Sprague EA, Kelley JL, Nerem RM. The pathogenesis of atherosclerosis: An overview. Clin Cardiol 1991; 14(Suppl I):1-16.
20.   Davies MJ, Woolf N. Atherosclerosis: What is it and why does it occur? Br Heart J 1993; 69(Suppl I):S3-S11.
21.   Poston R, Haskard D, Coucher J, Gall N, Johnson R. Expression of intercellular adhesion molecule-1 in atherosclerotic plaques. Am J Pathol 1992; 140:665-673.
22.   Hansson GK. Immune and inflammatory mechanisms of monocyte recruitment and accumulation. Br Heart J 1993; 69(Suppl):59-S29.
23.   Rabbani L, Loscalzo J. Recent observations on the role of hemostatic determinants in the development of the atherothrombotic plaque. Atherosclerosis 1994; 105:1-7.
24.   Roberts WC. Diffuse extent of coronary atherosclerosis in fatal coronary artery disease. Am J Cardiol 1990; 90:1614-1621.
25.   Falk E. Coronary Thrombosis: Pathogenesis and clinical manifestations. Am J Cardiol 1991;68:28B-35B.
26.   Falk E. Morphologic features of unstable atherothrombotic plaques underlying acute coronary syndromes. Am J Cardiol 1989; 63:114E-120E.
27.   Gertz SD, Roberts WC. Hemodynamic shear force in rupture of coronary arterial atherosclerotic plaques. Am J Cardiol. 1990; 66: 1368-1372.
28.   Stary HC. Evolution and progression of atherosclerotic lesions in coronary arteries of children and young adults. Arteriosclerosis 1989; 9(Suppl I):I19-I32.30.
29.   Davies MJ. A macro and micro view of coronary vascular insult in ischemic heart disease. Circulation 1990; 82(Suppl II):II38-II46.
30.   Falk E. Plaque rupture with severe preexisting stenosis precipitating coronary thrombosis: characteristics of coronary atherosclerotic plaques underlying fatal occlusive thrombi. Br Heart J 1983; 50:127-134.
31.   Richardson P, Davies M, Born G. Influence of plaque configuration and stress distribution on fissuring of coronary atherosclerotic plaques. Lancet. 1989; 2:941-44.
32.   Falk E, Shah PK, Fuster V. Coronary plaque rupture. Circulation. 1995; 92:657-671.

33. Fernandez-Ortiz A, Badimon J, Falk E, Fuster V, Meyer B, Mailhac A, Weng D, Shah PK, Badimon L. Characterization of the relative thrombogenicity of atherosclerotic plaque components: implications for consequences of plaque rupture. J Am Coll Cardiol. 1994; 23:1562-1569.
34. Wilcox JN, Smith KM, Schwartz SM, Gordon D. Localization of tissue factor in normal vessel wall and in the atherosclerotic plaque. Proc Natl Acad Sci USA 1989; 86:2839-2843.
35. Annex BH, Denning SM, Channon KM, Sketch MH Jr, Stack RS, Morrisey JH, Peters KG. Differential expression of tissue factor protein in directional atherectomy specimens from patients with stable and unstable coronary syndromes. Circulation 1995; 91:619-622.
36. Marmur J.D, Thiruvikraman SV, Fyfe BS, Guha A, Sharma SH, Ambrose JH, Fallon JT, Nemerson Y, Taubman M. The identification of active tissue factor in human coronary atheroma. Circ. In press 1966.
37. Toschi V, Gallo R, Lettino M, Fallon JT, Fernandez-Ortiz A, Badimon L, Chesebro JH, Nemerson Y, FusterV,Badimon JJ. Tissue Factor Modulates the Thrombogenicity of Human Atherosclerotic Plaque. Circulation 1997; 95:594-599.
38. Davies MJ, Thomas AC. Plaque fissuring. The cause of acute myocardial infarction, sudden death, ischemic death, and crescendo angina. Br. Heart J. 1985; 53:363-367.
39. Falk E. Morphologic features of unstable atherothrombotic plaques underlying acute coronary syndromes. Am J Cardiol 1990; 63:114E-120E.
40. Falk E. Coronary thrombosis: Pathogenesis and clinical manifestations. Am J Cardiol 1991; 68:28B-35B
41. Falk E. Why do plaques rupture?. Circulation 1992; 86: (Suppl III) 30-42.
42. Ambrose J. Nembaum D. Alexopoulos D. Angiographic progression of coronary artery disease and the development of myocardial infarction. J Am Coll Cardiol 1988; 12:56-62.
43. Little WC. Constantinescu M, Applegate RJ et al. Can coronary angiography predict the site of a subsequent myocardial infarction in patients with mild to moderate coronary artery disease? Circulation 1988; 78:1157-1166.
44. Levin D, Fallon JT. Significance of the angiographic morphology of localized coronary stenosis. Circulation 1982; 66:316-320.
45. Brown B, Gallery C, Badger R et al. Incomplete lysis of thrombus in the moderate underlying atherosclerotic   plaque during intracoronary infusion of streptokinase for acute myocardial infarction. Circulation 1986; 73:653-661.
46. Falk E. Unstable angina with fatal outcome: Dynamic coronary thrombosis leading to infarction and/or sudden death. Circulation 1985; 71:699-708.
47. Constantinides P. Plaque fissures in human coronary thrombosis, J Atheroscl. Res. 1966; 6:1-17.
48. Ornish D, Brown SE, Scherwitz LW. Can lifestyle changes reverse coronary artery disease? The Lifestyle Heart Trial. Lancet 1990; 336:129-133.
49. Brown G, Albers JJ, Fischer LD, et al. Regression of coronary artery disease as a result of intensive lipid lowering therapy in men with high levels of apolipoprotein B. N Engl J Med 1990; 336:129-133.
50. Frick M, Elo O, Haapa K, Heinonen O, Heimsalmi P, Helo P and the rest of the Helsinky Heart Study investigstors. Primary prevention trial with gemfibrozil in middle-aged men with dyslipemia. Safety of treatment, changes in risk factors, and incidence of coronary heart disease. N Engl J Med 1987; 317:1237-1245.
51. Blankenhorn DH, Nessim SA, Johnson RL. Beneficial effects of combined colestipol-niacin therapy on coronary atherosclerosis and coronary venous bypass grafts. JAMA 1987; 257:3233-3240.
52. Cashin-Hemphill L, Mack WJ, Pogoda JM, et al. Beneficial effects of colestipolniacin on coronary atherosclerosis. JAMA 1987; 257:3233-3240.
53. Buchwald H, Varco RI, Matts JP, et al. Effect of partial ileal bypass surgery on mortality and morbidity from coronary heart disease in patients with hyperlipidemia. N Engl J Med 1990; 323:946-955.
54. Watts GF, Lewis B, Brunt JN, et al. Effects on coronary artery disease of lipid-lowering diet, or diet plus cholestyramine in the St Thomas atherosclerosis regression study (STARS). Lancet 1992; 339:563-569.
55. Waters D, Higginson L, Gladstone P, Kimball B, Le May M, L'Esperance. Effects of monotherapy with an HMG-CoA reduce inhibitor on the progression of coronary atherosclerosis as assessed by serial quantitative arteriography. The Canadian Coronary Atherosclerosis Intervention Trial. Circulation. 1994; 89:959-968.
56. Badimon JJ, Badimon L, Fuster V. Regression of atherosclerotic lesions by high density lipoprotein plasma fraction in the cholesterol-fed rabbit. J Clin Invest. 1990; 85:1234-1241.
57. Scandinavian Simvastatin Survival Study Group. Randomised trial of cholesterol lowering in 4444 patien ts with coronary heart disease: the Scandinavian Simvastatin Survival Study (4S). Lancet. 1994;344:1383-1389.
58. Shepherd J, Cobbe SM, Ford I et al. Prevention of coronary heart disease with pravastatin in men with hypercholesterolemia. N Engl J Med 1995; 333:1301-1307.

59. Sacks FM, Pfeffer MA, Moye LA, Rouleau JL, Rutherford JD, Cole TG, Brown L, Warnica JW, Arnold JM, Wun CC, Davis Br, Braunwald E. The effect of pravastatin on coronary events after myocardial infarction in patients with average cholesterol levels. Cholesterol and Recurrent Events Trial, N Engl J Med, 1996; 335:1001-1009.60.

60. Byington RP, Jukema JW, Salonen JT. Reduction in cardiovascular events during pravastatin therapy. Circulation 1995; 92:2419-2425.

61. Cambien F, Costerousse 0, Tiret L, Poitier 0, Lecerf L, Gonzales MF, Evans A, Arveiler D, Cambou JP, Luc 6, Rakotovao R, Ducimetiere P, Soubrier F, Alhenc- Gelas F. Plasma level and gene polymorphism of angiotensin-converting enzyme in relation to myocardial infarction. Circulation. 1994; 90:669-676.

62. Yusuf S, Pepine CJ, Garces C, Pouleur H, Salem D, Kostis J, Benedict C, Rousseau M, Bourassa M, Pitt B. Effect of enalapril on myocardial infarction and unstable angina in patients with low ejection fractions. Lancet. 1992; 340:1173-1178.

63. Pfeffer MA, Braunwald E, on behalf of SAVE investigators. Effect of captopril on mortality and morbidity in patients with left ventricular dysfunction after myocardial infarction. N Engl J Med. 1992; 327:669-677.

64. Rutherford J, Pfeffer M, Moyt L, Davies B, Flaker G, Kowey P, Lamas G, Miller HS, Packer M, Rouleau J, Braunwaid E, on behalf of the SAVE Investigators. Effects of captopril on ischemic events after myocardial infarction: results of the Survival and Ventricular Enlargement trial. Circulation. 1994; 90:1731-1738.

65. The SOLVD investigators: Effect of enalapril on survival in patients with reduced left ventricular ejection fractions and congestive heart failure. N Engl J Med 1991; 325:293-298.

66. The SOLVD investigators: Effects of enalapril on mortality and the development of heart failure in asymptomatic patients with reduced left ventricular ejection fractions. N Engl J Med. 1992; 327:685-670.

67. Lonn EM, Yusuf S, Jha P, Montague TJ, Teo KK, Benedict CR, Pitt B. Emerging role of angiotensin-converting enzyme inhibitors in cardiac and vascular protection. Circulation. 1994; 90:2056-2069.

68. Hodis HN, Mack WJ, LaBree L, Hemphill LC, Azen SP. Natural antioxidant vitamins reduce coronary artery lesion progression as assessed by sequential coronary angiography. J Am Coll Cardiol. 1994; 23(Suppl A):481A. Abstract.

69. Gaziano JM. Antioxidant vitamins and coronary artery disease risk. Am J Med. 1994; 97:(Suppl 3A):3A-18-3A-21.

70. Walldius G, Erikson U, Olsson AG, Bergstrand L, Hadell K, Johansson J, Kaijser L, Lassvik C, Molgaard J, Nilsson S, SchäferElinder L, Stenport G, Holme 1. The effect of probucol on femoral atherosclerosis: The Probucol Quantitative Regression Swedish Trial (PQRST). Am J Cardiol. 1994; 74:875-883.

71. Byers T, Perry G. Dietary carotenes, vitamin C, and vitamin E as protective antioxidants in human cancers. Annu Rev Nutr 1992; 12:139-159

72. ha P, Flather M, Lonn E, Farkouh M, Yusuf S. The antioxidant vitamins and cardiovascular disease: a critical review of epidemiologic and clinical trial data. Ann Intern Med 1995; 123:860-872

73. Hennekens CH, Buring JE, Manson JE et al. Lack of effect of long-term supplementation with beta carotene on the incidence of malignant neoplasma and cardiovascular disease. N Engl J Med 1996;3 34:1145-1149.

74. Omenn GS, Goodman GE, Thornquist MD et al. Effects of a combination of beta carotene and vitamin A on lung cancer and cardiovascular disease. N Engl J Med1996; 334:1150-1155.

75. Kushi LH, Folsom AR, Prineas RJ, Mink PJ, Wu Y, Bostick RM. Dietary antioxidant vitamins and death from coronary heart disease in postmenopausal women. N Engl J Med 1996; 334:1156-1162.

76. Stephens NG, Parsons A, Scofield PM et al. Randomised controlled trial of vitamin E in patients with coronary disease: Cambridge Heart Antioxidant Study (CHAOS). Lancet 1996; 374:781-786.

77. Greenberg ER, Sporn MB. Antioxidant Vitamins, Cancer, and Cardiovascular Disease. Editorial. N Engl J Med 1996; 334 Number 18.

78. Stamper MJ, Colditz GA, Willett WC, Manson JE, Rosner B, Speizer FE, HennekensCHPostmenopausal estrogen therapy and cardiovascular disease: ten year follow-up from the nurses' healt study. N Engl J Med. 1991; 325:756-762.

79. Shahar E, Folsom AR, Salomaa VV, Stinson VL, McGovern PG, Shimakawa T, Chambless LE, WiKK for the atheroslerosis Risk in Communities (ARIC) Study Investigators. Relation of Hormone-Replacement Therapy to Measures of Plasma Fibrinolytic Activity. Circulation 1996; 93:1970-1975.

80. Jonas MA, Oates JA, Ockene J, Hennekens CH. Statement on smoking and cardiovascular disease for health care professionals. American Heart Association Medical/Scientific Statement. Circulation. 1992; 86:1664-1669.

81. Lichtlen PR, Nikutta P, Jost S, Deckers J, Wiese B, Rafflenbeul W, the INTACT Study Group. Anatomical progression of coronary artery disease in humans as seen by prospective, repeated, quantitated coronary angiography: relation to clinical events and risk factors. Circulation. 1992; 86:828-838.

82. Waters D, Higginson L, Gladstone P, Boccuzzi S, Cook T, Lespérance J. Smoking accelerates the progression of coronary atherosclerosis as assessed by serial quantitative coronary arteriography. Circulation. 1993; 88(suppl 1):I-344. Abstract.

83. Celermajer DS, Sorensen KE, Bull C, Robinson J, Deanfield JE. Endothelium-dependent dilation in the systemic arteries of asymptomatic subjects relates to coronary risk factors and their interaction. J Am Coll Cardiol. 1994; 24:1468-1474.

84. Kjekshus JK. Importance of heart rate in determining betablocker efficacy in acute and long-term acute myocardial infarction intervention trials. Am J Cardiol. 1986; 57(suppl F):43F-49F.

85. Wright RA, Flapan AD, Alberta KG, Ludlam CA, Fox KA. Effects of captopril therapy on endogenous fibrinolysis in men with recent, uncomplicated myocardial infarction. J Am Coll Cardiol. 1994; 24:67-73.

86. ACE Inhibitors use in patients with myocardial infarction. Summary of evidence from clinical trials. Circulation 1995; 92:3132-3137.

COLOR PLATES

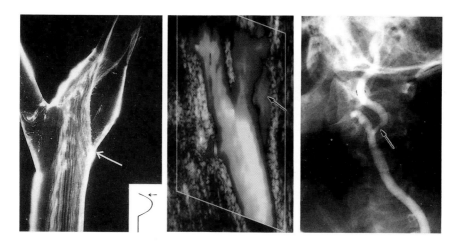

Bassiouny, *Figure 1. Model flow study of carotid bifurcation (a) During the ascending phase of systole, flow departs from it's laminar profile along the outer wall of this carotid sinus creating a recirculation region where wall shear stress is relatively low. In vivo color duplex imaging of a normal carotid bifurcation demonstrate this zone of flow reversal (blue area) (b). This represents the susceptible human carotid bifurcation sinus region for plaque formation (c).*

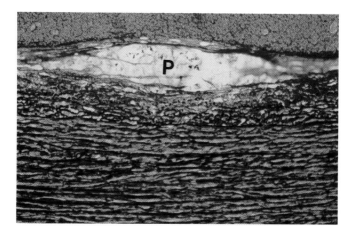

Bassiouny, *Figure 3. Minimal early atherosclerotic intimal thickening characterized by the accumulation of lipid containing foam cells (P) is noted within a narrow fibrocellular layer of intimal thickening.*

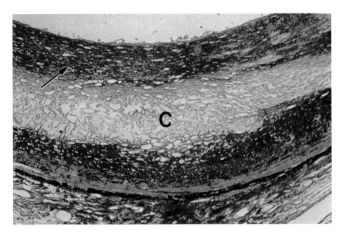

Bassiouny, *Figure 4. Segregation of a confluent lipid core © by subendothelial fibrocellular reactive thickening. A similar reaction is observed in the underlying media.*

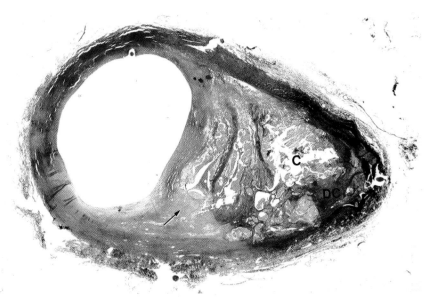

Bassiouny, *Figure 5. Advanced proximal internal carotid plaque with features of structural and compositional complexity. There are regions of lipid core formation (c), with apparent juxta medial fibrosis. (arrow) Degenerative tissue changes such as dystrophic calcification (DC) is also evident.*

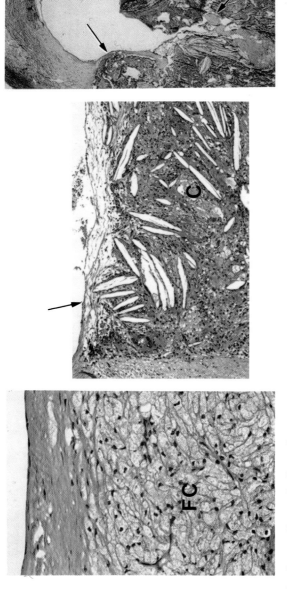
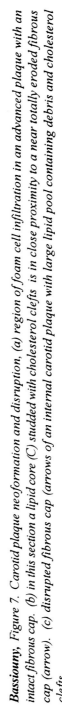

Bassiouny, Figure 7. *Carotid plaque neoformation and disruption. (a) region of foam cell infiltration in an advanced plaque with an intact fibrous cap. (b) in this section a lipid core (C) studded with cholesterol clefts is in close proximity to a near totally eroded fibrous cap (arrow). (c) disrupted fibrous cap (arrows of an internal carotid plaque with large lipid pool containing debris and cholesterol clefts.*

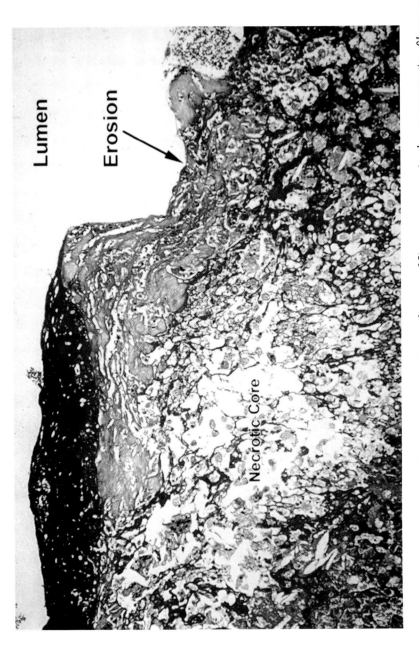

Bassiouny, *Figure 9. Photomicrograph of a histologic section (magnification x 25) in a symptomatic plaque representing fibrous cap thinning and erosion with exposure of the necrotic core to the lumen.*

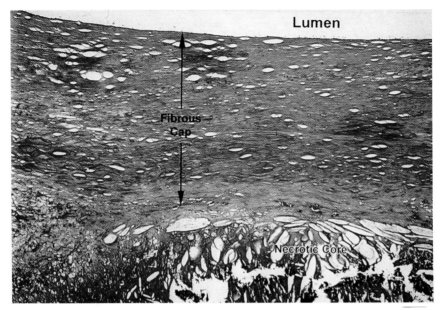

Bassiouny, *Figure 10. Photomicrograph (magnification x 15) illustrating a well developed fibrous cap isolating the plaque necrotic core from the lumen in an asymptomatic plaque.*

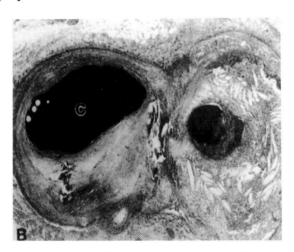

Badimon, *Figure 2. Histological illustration showing the different morphology of the coronary atherosclerotic plaques obtained in the same individual. The one on the left is a stable plaque while the one on the right is a disrupted plaque. Note the blue staining on the plaque indicative of its high content in fibrous tissue. The disrupted one shows a lipid-rich central core separated from the lumen by a thin fibrous cap; typical characteristics of the so-called "vulnerable plaques" (c-central lumen) (Courtesy of Dr. E. Falk).*

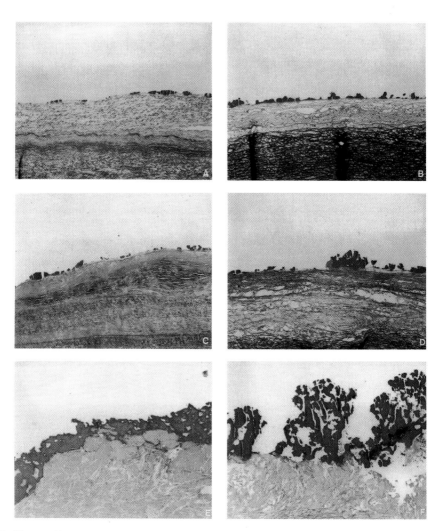

Badimon, *Figure 3. Representative photomicrographs from the different types of substrates exposed to flowing blood. Longitudinal sections of an intimal segment of human atherosclerotic plaque showing: A, right cellular layer without lipid infiltration. B, form cell rich matrix. C, collagen-rich matrix. D, collagen-poor matrix without cholesterol crystals. E and F, a cellular collagen poor soft core with abundant cholesterol crystals. Thrombus formed on the surfaces is stained in red. Note the formation of larger thrombi on atheromatous core (E and F). Trichromex 100 (from **ref.** 35)*

SECTION   II

DETECTION AND MONITORING OF ATHEROSCLEROSIS

VALIDITY AND REPRODUCIBILITY OF B-MODE ULTRASOUND IN IMAGING CAROTID INTIMA MEDIA THICKNESS

Michele Mercuri, M.D., Ph.D., Rong Tang, M.D. and M. Gene Bond, Ph.D.

Bowman Gray School of Medicine of Wake Forest University
Winston-Salem, North Carolina U.S.A.

Contents

I. INTRODUCTION

B-mode ultrasound imaging of carotid arteries was first introduced by Olinger in 1969 (1). Since then, this method has been refined and is widely used in all settings of the medical field from basic science to patients' care. The early reports focused on the potential of a noninvasive method which could couple in short sequence hemodynamic and morphologic information. The latest reports suggest that this methodology, in addition to providing prospective and serial information on how arterial wall and luminal dimension changes, can generate important insights into endothelial function and vascular remodeling.

II. RATIONALE FOR DEVELOPING NON INVASIVE VASCULAR IMAGING

Results from the International Atherosclerosis Project (IAP) (2) provided the largest database ever acquired about the pathobiology of human atherosclerosis. The IAP research outcomes opened a window of opportunities for preventing cardiovascular disease. The IAP investigators together with clinical epidemiologists posed the need for new diagnostic techniques suitable for in vivo investigations of atherosclerosis in large populations of high risk but still asymptomatic subjects.

Angiographic imaging of coronary, carotid and femoral arteries were extensively used and important data gathered to the scientific community. However, it is relevant to say that the rapid development of quantitative ultrasonography is based on its value as a surrogate for coronary artery disease, its direct relationship to cerebrovascular diseases and the possibility of prospectively studying the effects of risk factors management as inferred by changes in plaques present in peripheral vessels (see following chapter).

Noninvasive diagnosis of peripheral arteries can be accomplished with ultrasound devices (i.e., Doppler and/or imaging), magnetic resonance imaging and oculo-plethysmography. However, ultrasound methods have been leading the way and are the most widely used. The reasons for this success are several, but mostly because of inexpensiveness, reliability and versatility. In the area of vascular disease prevention, where the target population is largely made of young adult asymptomatic at high cardiovascular risk, ultrasound imaging is very widely used. Its way to the top passed through several testing obstacles including definition of predictive vascular endpoints, validity and reproducibility.

III. DEFINITIONS OF VASCULAR ENDPOINTS

Originally, ultrasound imaging developed as an aid to improve the ability of Doppler velocimetry in quantitating the lumen dimension. In fact it is well known that Doppler diagnosis functions in quite large categorical classes of vessel stenosis. While this is the case when the question is whether the patient's neurological symptoms may have a carotid origin, it falls short in all cases when one wants to have a more precise quantification of the extent and severity of the arterial disease or after the realization that vascular events are not necessarily associated with large and stenosing plaques. In consequence, ultrasound imaging techniques were more frequently used in subjects with early stages of the disease and/or to define the plaque morphologic characteristics. Under these circumstances, ultrasound imaging protocols were redesigned to maximize their imaging potential shifting the main interest from the lumen to studying the wall and its morphology (Figure 1).

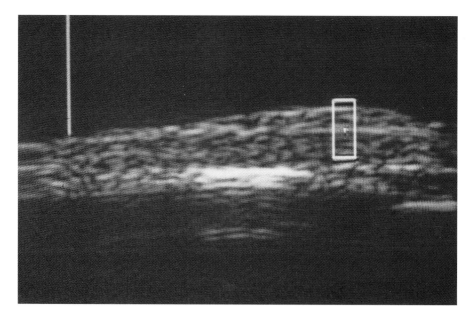

Figure 1. In vitro B-mode ultrasound of human thoracic aorta imaged in a water bath (37°C) with a 8 MHZ probe. The long bar indicates the left margin of an arterial segment with no evidence of atherosclerosis. The box (1.5 x 0.5 mm) shows an early atherosclerotic plaque. The central dot indicates the boundary between thickened intima (0.85 mm) and normal media. The bottom margin of the box is just above the ultrasonic interface between the arterial media and adventitia. Ultrasound imaging provides quantitative information about tissue texture.

Researchers developed several measures of extent and severity of vessel wall alterations based on arterial thickness (3). Early on, patients and/or subjects were classified according to large classes of thicknesses into cases and controls. Then, composite measures of extent and severity of carotid thickness were proposed in order to increase the analytical and prognostic power of ultrasound based risk factor stratifications. Lately, research with ultrasound imaging is being used to estimate plaque areas, lesion volumes, 3 dimensional reconstruction and to quantify vascular reactivity in peripheral arteries and test hypotheses related to endothelial dysfunction.

IV. VALIDITY

In the late 1970s and early 1980s important studies were designed and conducted to determine whether B-mode ultrasound imaging could be used to image validly and reliably the arterial wall. The first information regarding cross correlation between ultrasound and pathology was probably reported by Bond et al. (4). In this study, real time imaging measurements of human common carotid cross sections were compared to the ones obtained by histologic assessment. The initial coefficient of correlation was reported as a disappointing 0.30. Nonetheless, this observation prompted the interest of several investigators mostly because pointed at ways to reduce the variability and improve the internal validity of noninvasive and real time imaging of arteries. In fact, a few years later, Pignoli reported better results by improving image acquisition and interpretation (5).

A. Animal Experimentations

A second set of other preliminary, but critical observations were reported by Bond et al. (6). These experiments were designed to gain information on variables affecting the quality of images to improve wall measurements and to better define correlations with established imaging modalities. A colony consisting of 28 adult male Macaca Fascicularis (Cynomolgus) monkeys was used to investigate whether various degrees of atherosclerosis could be studied with ultrasound. Macacas were chosen because lesions resembling human plaques rapidly develop in the presence of hypertension (induced by aortic coarctation) and/or diet induced hypercholesterolemia. These animals were followed up for 26 months, and before necropsy, underwent aortic and carotid B-mode ultrasound (Horizon Research Laboratories, Inc., Fort Lauderdale, FL) and angiographic examinations to compare different vascular imaging modalities. Following necropsy, arteries were processed histologically to determine the ultrasound ability to image plaques. The results of these experiments showed that ultrasound can provide imaging information to measure both arterial lumen diameters and wall thicknesses. The correlation coefficients between ultrasound and pathology were 0.41 and 0.42 for lumen dimension and wall thickness respectively. Reproducibility was better for lumen (r=0.81) than for wall (0.47) measurements. However, these experiments were critical steps towards the definition of the criteria to be considered for developing a quantitative protocol which would have allowed the application of B-mode ultrasound in prospective investigations. In fact the experiments' findings pointed at a series of factors which significantly influence the feasibility of serial measurements of arterial characteristics, such as the specific settings of the ultrasound system, the sampling methodology to select the arterial segments to choose the follow-up, the need for identifying specific anatomical landmarks, and most importantly strengths and weaknesses of endpoints such as the arterial wall thickness and the lumen dimension.

B. The NIH Multicenter (US) Validation Study

Some of these issues were further explored within the NIH sponsored US Multicenter Validation Study (7-9). This comprehensive project included the participation of researchers from different areas of expertise, i.e., basic science, neurology, radiology, and surgery, and provided an extremely useful in depth investigation over the issues raised by the early laboratory and animal investigations. The consensus was that serial measurements of the arterial wall and diameter could be reliably undertaken using B-mode ultrasound. Though, arteriography seemed to be superior in quantifying lumen dimension, B-mode offered significant advantages in determining the plaque size and in providing information on tissue structure. In addition, these investigations provided critical information regarding interlaboratory standardization, and the elements for properly evaluating measurement variability.

C. The Baylor College of Medicine Study on Atherosclerosis Progression

Following the preliminary investigations aimed at determining the potential use of noninvasive ultrasound imaging systems with animal model of atherosclerosis, a pilot, but critical experiment was undertaken by Insull et al. at the Baylor College of Medicine, Houston, TX (10). This clinical trial, though small, impacted tremendously on the future development of the protocols for interventional clinical trials of atherosclerosis using B-mode ultrasound imaging. The goals for this investigation were to determine whether B-mode ultrasound imaging could be used to demonstrate plaque progression, and to define which arterial endpoint, i.e., lumen or wall thickness, should be used in prospective investigations of atherosclerosis. The carotid arteries of 28 cardiovascular asymptomatic men (mean age 55 years, range 39-60) with moderate to severe hypercholesterolemia (mean LDL-cholesterol 185 mg/dL, LDL/HDL 4.16) were continuously examined for 16 months with a 10 MHZ B-mode ultrasound system (Horizon Research Laboratories Inc., Fort Lauderdale, FL). The ultrasound protocol included multiple interrogations at the single thickest plaque site. The ultrasound examinations aimed at defining the thickness of the plaque measured as the total wall thickness, i.e., intima-media-adventitia thickness and the lumen dimension. Follow-up scans were performed after 6 and 12 months. The follow up was supposed to continue regularly for up to 2 to 3 years. However, new findings providing strong support to the association of elevated LDL-cholesterol and cardiovascular morbidity and mortality, and the release of new recommendations to treat patients with hypercholesterolemia, prompted an early stop of the investigation and a final scan was performed about 16 months after the initial examination. The results show that B-mode imaging could reliably demonstrate the progression of the plaque (from 1.47 to 1.92 mm) and the parallel reduction in the lumen dimension (from 6.02 to 5.65 mm) (Figure 2). One of the findings reported was also suggesting that smaller lesions progress more rapidly than the larger ones.

This study was the first to report the ability of ultrasound imaging to describe noninvasively the natural progression of carotid plaque. This report also impacted on the extrapolation of the seminal work published by Pignoli et al. (11), and the ideation of larger and more sophisticated attempts to determine whether medical intervention, i.e., lipid lowering and blood pressure drugs, could affect the progression of asymptomatic and early stages of atherosclerosis.

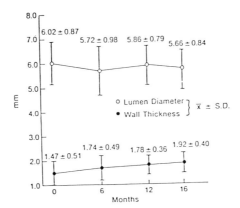

Figure 2. B-mode ultrasound monitoring of carotid artery plaques over 16 months. Measurements of carotid wall thickness and lumen diameter performed at a single site in each of 28 subjects. Thicknesses are in mm and data monthly averages are mean ± S.D. From reference 10.

D. The Pignoli's Experiment

Though important, all the experiments above had a common weakness, they lacked a solid interpretation of the arterial wall as imaged by ultrasound. This hole was filled by critical experiments designed by Pignoli et al. (11).

Pignoli started from the observation that ultrasound images the arterial wall as a sequence of echogenic lines. Secondly, he made the assumption that while intimal and medial acoustic impedance is relatively constant and similar to the reflection coefficient of muscles, echoes are generated by the change in density occurring at tissue interfaces (Figure 3). In addition, Pignoli et al. focused their attention to a "double line" pattern that seemed to be commonly present both *in vitro* and *in vivo* when longitudinally imaging tubular structure similar to non diseased common carotid arteries or any other major elastic artery (class A). They also observed that this pattern was less frequent in presence of obvious diseased walls (class B), i.e. , typical in 56%, complex in 24% and absent in 20%. Insertion and dissection experiments were performed to identify specific histologic structures, i.e. , the boundary between lumen and arterial surface and the boundary between medial and adventitial tunicae. Acquisition and measurements of the arterial wall with quantitative ultrasound imaging in both *in vitro* and *in vivo* experiments prove that the linear distance between the two echogenic lines expressing the double line pattern were significantly close to the thickness of the intima plus media as measured by histology (r=0.76 and 0.82, class A and B respectively) and gross pathology (r=0.87 and 0.93). Pignoli's work also provided significant insights into the problem of measurement reproducibility that became later the focus of all protocols used in interventional clinical trials.

Pignoli's interpretation received tremendous attention, referenced widely and used very extensively to design protocols for observational and interventional clinical trials trials. This piece of work went unchallenged for several years not because was superficially accepted by the scientific community, but because was timely, scientifically sound and extremely original. However, most recently Gamble et al. (12) presented the results of a study intended to replicate Pignoli's interpretation and challenging some of his conclusions. Specifically, Gamble confirmed that B-mode ultrasound is a valid method to measure the arterial wall thickness, but his group data favor a closer correlation between histologic wall assessment and intimal-medial-adventitial thickness. In a separate report, Wong et al. (13), confirmed Pignoli's interpretation, and additionally provided data suggesting that low frequency B-mode ultrasound (7-10 MHZ) cannot be used to measure individual arterial tunicae. Wong presented results showing that while the medial tunica is accurately measured by ultrasound, intima and adventitia are usually overestimated, though this variance is not significant especially when imaging the far wall. Alternatively, Mercuri et al. (14), reported good results also for near wall measurements, but pointed out to extreme differences caused by experimental settings and technical specs of mechanical and digital imagers (15). Subsequently, Hodges et al. (16), proposed to simplify the measurement process by shifting the interest from IMT to the total wall thickness. Hodges argument being that total wall thickness is easier to measure and retain the same predictive power as IMT. The issue confronting different schools about validity of near vs. far wall measurements created controversies and is still unresolved. However, consensus exists that while theoretically it may be incorrect to measure the near wall, available data from several different laboratories provide a solid argument against the theory. In fact, near wall measurements increase the detecting and predicting power of ultrasound imaging and provide a better description of a volumetric phenomenon like atherosclerosis (17).

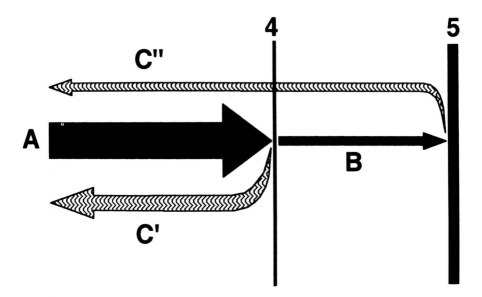

Figure 3. B-mode ultrasound images the vessel wall as a double line pattern. An incident beam (A) encounters the arterial surface (4), and because of the density differential, is partially reflected back to the transducer (C'). This signal provides imaging information (strength and location) of the ultrasonic interface between lumen and arterial surface (near wall or interface 4). The residual energy of the ultrasound beam allows further traveling into the vessel wall (B). This beam is further reflected back in quantities that are proportional to the density of the biologic structure, and provide imaging information about tissue texture. When B encounters the interface between the arterial media and the adventitia, a second major attenuation (or reflection) occurs (C") and the image of the far wall or interfaces 5 is displayed on the ultrasound monitor.

V.   QUANTITATIVE METHODS

Early ultrasound imaging protocols were very clinical oriented and relied very little on specific sampling methods. In fact, as described above, ultrasound imaging was mostly used to improve detection of significant disease in neurologic patients. Semiquantitative methods were first applied to ultrasound imaging to relate risk factors to severity of extracranial carotid diseases (3). Initially, and before Pignoli's work, measures of arterial walls were made manually from the device monitor and relied heavily on physicians' interpretation. Therefore, the early data were extremely operator dependent and held large interlaboratory variations. However, Bond and Pignoli first and later the NIH (US)

Multicenter Validation Study provided ample ground for a more objective image interpretation, to reduce interlaboratory variations, and to set criteria for a more quantitative approach.

One of the first results achieved by the NIH (US) Multicenter Validation Study was the acknowledgment that to perform a meaningful ultrasound study a written protocol must be available. This protocol must contain specific procedures to standardize instrument setting, operators' training and monitoring, scanning and sampling methodology, image interpretation and wall thickness measurements, and last, but not least, effective quality control procedures. The first standardized protocol released to researchers interested in noninvasive vascular investigations was the ultrasound protocol of the Atherosclerosis Risk In Community Study (ARIC) (18). ARIC is an ongoing observational investigation in which ultrasound imaging is heavily used. The ARIC ultrasound protocol resulted from the collaborative effort of several researchers involved in early methodological investigations and focused on sampling method to acquire data prospectively (standardization) and make the image interpretation and thickness quantification as objective as possible. The key features of the ARIC protocol are: the use of the same ultrasound instrument in all the centers involved in the investigation; centralized training and continuous monitoring for all operators (sonographers and readers); ultrasound core laboratory where image interpretation and quantification are performed using semiautomatic image processing reading stations; standardization of ultrasound imaging by restricting wall measurements to the carotid bifurcation area (distal common, bifurcation and proximal internal) defined by two anatomical landmarks: the initial dilation of the bulb and the tip of the flow divider; routine assessment of reproducibility by randomly repeating examinations and readings. The standardization by the ARIC group is widely accepted and followed worldwide. A few variations of the ARIC protocol exist, but are mostly confined to the number of arterial projections recorded and the number of walls considered for the analyses. In particular, many of the epidemiological studies use a simplified protocol in which preselected projections of the vessel wall are used (i.e. , anterior, lateral and posterior-lateral) while measurements are restricted to the far wall of the distal common. These features are usually adopted to reduce the time required for examining the patients who in addition to vascular ultrasound are screened with extensive questionnaires, blood work and several other diagnostic tests. The protocols used in interventional controlled clinical trials adopt a more extensive imaging approach which maximize the area investigated with ultrasound by producing a circumpherencial scans covering as much of the arterial surface as possible (19). In addition, arterial thickness is measured in up to 12 walls including the near and far wall of the distal common, bifurcation/bulb and proximal internal carotid artery.

The most recent protocols include the use of image processing stations equipped with edge detection softwares that use pixel intensity algorithms to identify ultrasonic interfaces and automatically calculate intima media thicknesses at prespecified discrete arterial segments. These softwares are becoming standard and allowed the acquisition of large amount of information coupled with very effective data management.

VI.   REPRODUCIBILITY

The concept of measurement reproducibility in ultrasound imaging has evolved as these protocols are used more frequently in large epidemiologic studies and controlled clinical trials. In fact, while originally confined to small data sets and single laboratories, the application of vascular ultrasound protocol has extended to studies with several thousand patients followed for several years and frequent follow up visits. As a consequence, reproducibility has become an important variable in estimating the sample size for an investigation, conditions the model to be used for the statistical analyses, and is of critical importance to define the outcome of the trials.

Currently, definition of measurement reproducibility is a requirement for any meaningful study using B-mode ultrasonography. Traditionally, reproducibility is measured by repeating measurements of IMT in a quota of exams. In the past this activity has been confined to cross sectional determinations of differences between repeat measure of the outcome variable and expressed as a coefficient of variation and/or a coefficient of correlation. Crouse et al. (20) cited an estimate of reproducibility based on rescans performed on the same patients six months apart from each other resulting in a coefficient of 0.86. In the NIH (US) Multicenter Validation Study, O'Leary et al. (8) reported within reader coefficients of correlation of 0.72 to 0.77 and those between reader agreement from 0.48 and 0.65. However, the current standard index of reproducibility is the absolute difference between two estimates expressed in mm.

Major observational studies reported data on measurement reproducibility. However, because of the time and resources involved, these databases are usually limited to a small number of participants. Salonen et al. (21) performed a small, but dedicated reproducibility experiment focusing on intra and inter observer differences in examining the average maximal right and left far wall of the distal common carotid arteries. Ten subjects, randomly selected among middle-age eastern Finnish men participating in the Kuopio Ischemic Heart Disease Risk Factor Study (KIHD) (22), were examined three times by three sonographers. The mean far wall common carotid artery IMT was 1.08 mm (range 0.6 to 2.4 mm), the mean inter observer coefficient of variation was 10.5%, while the intra observer coefficient ranged between 5.41 to 5.77%. The absolute differences for the far wall of the common carotid IMT ranged between 0.06 to 0.09 mm. Persson et al. (23) reported an overall absolute difference of 0.09 mm in repeated measurements of the far wall of common carotid IMT in 134 asymptomatic subjects blindly examined by two sonographers-readers. In ARIC the average absolute differences between replicate scans of either right or left far common, bifurcation and internal carotid IMT ranged between 0.29 and 0.74. O'Leary et al. (24) reported baseline reproducibility data for the Cardiovascular Health Study (CHS). Reproducibility studies were performed to estimate the inter and intra sonographer, and inter reader variabilities. Maximum and mean IMTs were measured blindly twice for the distal common and proximal internal carotid arteries in over 100 subjects recruited in CHS. Mean and maximum IMTs for the common and the internal were 0.73, 0.83 and 1.28, 1.67 mm respectively. Absolute differences for the mean IMT in the common carotids were 0.18, 0.13 and 0.10mm (inter and intra sonographer, and inter reader). Respective figures for the internal carotid were 0.6, 0.66 and 0.4. Bots et al. (25) reported reproducibility information for the Rotterdam Study. Eighty subjects were randomly selected among the 1000 participants and examined twice within a 3 month period. Absolute differences were calculated between two replicate estimates of the far wall of the left and right common carotid IMT. Each measure was the mean of three quantitations. The right and left absolute differences for inter readers (n=75) and inter sonographers (n=77) were 0.04 and 0.069 mm.

Reproducibility data are routinely reported by all major controlled clinical trials. Mercuri et al. reported information for the Multicenter Isradipine Diuretic Atherosclerosis Study (MIDAS) (26). In MIDAS the quality control protocol called for repeat examinations and readings of all the baseline and final scans plus a quota of 20% of the semiannual interim examinations. Reproducibility was calculated for a number of ultrasound endpoints. The absolute differences in 883 patients for the mean maximum IMT (i.e. , the mean of up to 12 maximal thicknesses) for baseline intra and inter operator variability was 0.12 mm. This difference was 0.36 mm for the single maximum thickness.

Table 1. *Reproducibility of B-mode ultrasound measures of carotid intima media thickness in controlled studies or clinical trials.*

Reference	n. of pts	CCA	Bif	ICA	Mean Max
Salonen et al (21)	10	0.06-0.09[1][2]	-	-	-
Persson et al (23)	134	0.09[1]	-	-	-
O'Leary et al (24)	100	0.10-0.18[2]	-	0.4-0.7[2]	-
Bots et al (25)	80	0.04-0.07[1][2]	-	-	-
Mercuri et al (26)	883	0.11	0.21	0.11	0.12
Riley et al (27)	858	-	-	-	0.10-0.11[2]
Mercuri et al (28)	305	0.05	0.10	0.10	0.07
Mercuri et al (29)	1754	0.08	0.13	-	0.08

[1] Far wall only
[2] Ranges of means for intra-inter-operator variabilities

Similar figures, relative to the cross sectional assessment of variability, were reported during the 3 year study. The reproducibility of the Asymptomatic Carotid Artery Progression Study (ACAPS) was reported by Riley et al. (27). Baseline reproducibilities (absolute difference for within and between sonographer) for the mean maximum IMT in 858 paired examinations performed 1 month apart before randomization were 0.10 (r=0.79) and 0.11 (r=0.75) mm and stayed constant over the 3 year long study. Intra and inter reader variabilities were assessed by rereading 40 pairs. Absolute differences were 0.05 (r=0.95) and 0.09 (r=0.73) respectively. In the Carotid Atherosclerosis Italian ultrasound Study (CAIUS) (28), examinations and readings were repeated in all 305 patients at baseline, after 18 and 36 months of follow up. At baseline, the absolute differences in replicate quantitations for the mean maximum IMT was 0.07 mm (95th percentile 0.194 mm, r=0.85). Absolute differences were 0.07 (0.16 mm, r=0.86) and 0.08 (0.192, r=0.82) mm afterwards. Recently, quality control procedures and interim reproducibility data from the European Lacidipine Study on Atherosclerosis (ELSA) were presented (29). This large multinational clinical trial recruited more than 2,200 patients with hypertension. Initial data show that the mean absolute difference in measuring the mean maximum intima media thickness in 1754 replicate blind examinations and readings is 0.078 mm. This is the first ultrasound based study using a comprehensive assessment of measurement variability. The scientific protocol details specific and prospective quantitation of cross sectional and longitudinal variability. Therefore, the ELSA database will allow performing inferential analyses to asses the effect of measurement variability on outcome endpoints. This is a critical step to better define the predictive power of ultrasound endpoints on individual patient cardiovascular risk.

VII. SUMMARY

B-mode ultrasound imaging has been demonstrated to be a valid and reproducible noninvasive system to study the morphologic characteristics of the arterial wall. Quantitative protocols derived from animal, laboratory, autoptic and human studies have been refined to provide acceptable cross sectional and longitudinal measurements of carotid IMT. Quantitative ultrasonography requires careful decisions in term of instrumentation, operators' training and quality control procedures, however if the above is taken into consideration, this technique can be used with high confidence in large observational studies and in multinational-multicenter interventional clinical trials.

Acknowledgments

Our gratitude goes to Dr. Mariarita Pignatelli, Bowman Gray School of Medicine, Winston-Salem, USA. This work was supported in part by grants from the Italian Research Council and the Italian Ministry for Higher Education (MM).

References

1. Olinger CP: Ultrasonic Carotid Echoarteriography. Am J Radiology 1969;106:282-295
2. Solberg LA, McGarry PA, Moosy J, Strong JP, Tejada C, Laken AC: Severity of Atherosclerosis in Cerebral Arteries, Coronary Arteries, and Aortas. Ann NY Acad Sci 1968;149:956-973
3. Crouse JR, Thompson CJ: Evaluation of Methods for Quantifying Lumen Stenosis and Atherosclerosis. Circulation 1993;87(suppl. II):II-17,II-33
4. Bond MG, Riley WA, Barnes RW, Raduck JM, Ball MR: Validation Studies of a Noninvasive Real Time B Scan Imaging System. In:. Non Invasive Techniques for Assessment of Atherosclerosis in Peripheral, carotid and Coronary Arteries. Berson AS, Budinger TF, Ringquist I et al. (Eds.), Raven press, 1982:197
5. Pignoli P: Ultrasound B-mode Imaging for Arterial Wall Thickness Measurement. Atherosclerosis Rev 1984;12:177
6. Bond MG, Berson AS, Bryan FA: Ultrasound Imaging of Atherosclerotic Lesions in Arteries of Animals: Validity and Reproducibility. In: Atherosclerotic Plaques. Wissler RW (ed), Plenum Press, 1991, 17-26.

7.   Ricotta Jj, Bryan Fa, Bond Mg et al.: Multicenter Validation Study of Real-time (B-mode) Ultrasound, Arteriography, and Pathologic Examination. J Vasc Surg 1987;6:512.

8.   O'leary Dh, Bryan Fa, Goodison Mw et al.: Measurement Variability of Carotid Atherosclerosis: Real-time (B-mode) Ultrasonography and Angiography. Stroke 1987;18:1011.

9.   Schenk Ea, Bond Mg, Aretz Th et al.:. Multicenter Validation Study of Real-time Ultra-sonography, Arteriography, and Pathology: Pathologic Evaluation of Carotid Endarterectomy Specimens. Stroke 1989;119:289.

10.   Insull W jr, Bond MG, Wilmoth S, Fishel J, Herson J: Ultrasound Lesions of the Carotid Artery and Risk Factors in Men. In: S Glagov, Newman WP III, Schaffer SA: Pathobiology of the Human Atherosclerotic Plaque. Springer, New York, 1990, pp. 663-669

11.   Pignoli P, Tremoli E, Poli A, Oreste P, Paoletti R: Intimal Plus Medial Thickness of the Arterial Wall: A Direct Measurement With Ultrasound Imaging. Circulation 1986;74:1399-1406

12.   Gamble G, Beaumont B, Smith H et al.: B-mode Ultrasound Images of the Carotid Artery Wall: Correlation of Ultrasound With Histological Measurements. Atherosclerosis 1993;102:163-173

13.   Wong M, Edelstein J, Wollman J, Bond MG.: Ultrasonic-pathological comparison of the human arterial wall. Verification of intima-media thickness. Arterioscl Thromb 1993; 13:482-6.

14.   Mercuri M, Tang R, Bond MG: Validity and Reproducibility of B-Mode Ultrasound Imaging in Measuring the Near Wall (Abstract) Circulation 1991;84(suppl. II):II-541

15.   Nolsoe CP, Engel U, Karstrop S et al.,: The Aortic Wall: An in Vitro Study of the Double-Line Pattern in High Resolution US. Radiology 1990;175:387 (see letter)

16.   Hodges TC, Detmer PR, Dawson DL et al.: Ultrasound Determination of Total Arterial Wall Thickness. J Vasc Surg 1994;19:745-753

17.   Berglund GL: Minisymposium: Ultrasound in Clinical Trials of Atherosclerosis. Introduction. Journal of Internal Medicine 1994; 236: 551-553

18.   ARIC Investigators: The Atherosclerosis Risk in Communities (ARIC) Study: Design and Objectives. American Journal of Epidemiology 1989;129:687-702

19.   Mercuri M: Noninvasive Imaging Protocols to Detect and Monitor Carotid Atherosclerosis Progression. American Journal of Hypertension 1994; 7:23S-29S

20.   Crouse JR, Harpold GH, Kahl FR, Toole JF, McKinney WM: Evaluation of a Scoring System for Extracranial Carotid Atherosclerosis Extent with B-Mode Ultrasound. Stroke 1986;17:270-275

21.   Salonen R, Haapanen A, Salonen JT: Measurement of Intima Media Thickness of Common Carotid Arteries with High Resolution B-Mode Ultrasonography: Inter and Intra-observer Variability. Ultrasound Med Biol 1991-17:225-230

22.   Salonen JT, Salonen R.: Ultrasound B-mode imaging in observational studies of atherosclerotic progression. Circulation 1993;87 (suppl II):56-65.

23.   Persson J, Stavenow L, Wikstrand J et al.: Noninvasive Quantification of Atherosclerotic Lesions. Reproducibility of Ultrasonographic Measurement of Arterial Wall Thickness and Plaque Size. Arterioscler Thromb 1992;12:261-266

24.   O'Leary DH, Polak JF, Wolfson SK et al.: Use of Sonography to Evaluate Carotid Atherosclerosis in the Elderly. The Cardiovascular Health Study. Stroke 1991;22:1155-1163

25.   Bots ML, Breslau PJ, Briet Eet al.: Cardiovascular determinants of carotid artery disease. The Rotterdam Elderly Study. Hypertension 1992;19:717-20

26.   Mercuri M, Bond MG, Nichols FT, Carr AA, Flack JM, Byington R, Raines J.: Baseline Reproducibility of B-mode Ultrasound Imaging Measurements of Carotid Intima Media Thickness: The Multicenter Isradipine Diuretic Atherosclerosis Study (MIDAS). J Cardiovascular Diagnosis and Procedures 1993;11:241-255

27.   Riley WA, Barnes RW, Applegate WB et al.: Reproducibility of Noninvasive Ultrasonic Measurements of Carotid Atherosclerosis. The Asymptomatic Carotid Artery Plaque Study (ACAPS). Stroke 1992; 23:1062-1068.

28.   Mercuri M, Bond MG, Sirtori CR et al.: Pravastatin Reduces Carotid Intima media Thickness Progression in an Asymptomatic Hypercholesterolemic Mediterranean population. The Carotid Atherosclerosis Italian Ultrasound Study. Am J Med 1996;101:627-634

29.   Mercuri M, Tang R, Phillips RM, Bond MG: Ultrasound Protocol and Quality Control Procedures in the European Lacidipine Study on Atherosclerosis (ELSA). Blood Pressure 1996;5(Suppl. 4):20-23

ENDOTHELIAL FUNCTION AND NON-INVASIVE DETECTION AND QUANTIFICATION OF BRACHIAL ARTERY REACTIVITY

Rong Tang, M.D., Michele Mercuri, M.D., Ph.D. and M. Gene Bond, Ph.D.

Bowman Gray School of Medicine of Wake Forest University,
Winston-Salem, North Carolina   U.S.A.

Contents

I. Endothelium-dependent Vaso Relaxation, EDRF and NO

    A. EDRF

    B. Nitric Oxide and Its Physiology

        1. NO Release

        2. Shear-Stress-Induced release of NO by the Endothelium

        3. Cardiovascular Physiology of NO

II. Endothelial Dysfunction in Atherosclerosis

    A. Mechanism underlying Endothelial Dysfunction in Atherosclerosis

        1. Impaired NO Production

        2. Shortened NO Half-life

III. Detection and Quantification of Endothelial Dysfunction

    A. Systemic Nature of Endothelial Dysfunction

    B. Non-Invasive Assessment of Brachial Artery Vasoreactivity

        1. Vasodilation Test, Imaging and Data Acquisition

        2. Reproducibility

    C. Arterial reactivity and Atherogenesis

        1. Aging

        2. Estrogens

        3. Cigarette Smoking

        4. Hypercholesterolemia and Risk Factor Interaction

        5. Hypertension

        6. Diabetes Mellitus

        7. Evaluation of Therapeutic Effects

IV. Summary

I. ENDOTHELIUM-DEPENDENT VASO RELAXATION, EDRF AND NO

It has been found that endothelium-dependent arterial relaxation is impaired in various pathological conditions, such as hypercholesterolemia (1), atherosclerosis (2,3), or systemic hypertension (4). Before anatomical evidence of atherosclerosis, endothelial dysfunction may present an early event in the natural history of vascular disease. It has been observed that endothelial dysfunction correlated with the progression of atherosclerosis (2) and in addition, endothelium-dependent vessel relaxation is attenuated in the vessels even without angiographically or intravascular ultrasound detected lesions in patients at risk of atherosclerosis (5,6,7). Thus, endothelial dysfunction is the most sensitive marker of early atherosclerosis. Furthermore, *in vitro* and *in vivo* studies have demonstrated the link between endothelial dysfunction and impaired release of substances from endothelium, such as endothelium-derived relaxing factor (EDRF) and prostacyclin (8) which have anti-atherogenic properties and are responsible for regulation of vascular tone.

The recently developed method using B-mode ultrasound imaging to assess brachial vessel reactivity enables us to non-invasively evaluate endothelial function in various populations. This technique measures the change of the brachial artery diameter induced by the reactive hyperemia in the forearm. The increased shear stress stimulates endothelium to release EDRF that results in arterial dilation. Therefore, the change of brachial artery diameter depends on the release of EDRF, in other words, endothelial function.

A. EDRF

EDRF was first identified in vitro by Furchgott and Zawadzki in 1980 (9). They observed that acetylcholine constricted the arterial segment with a damaged endothelium, but relaxed the artery with an intact endothelium, and concluded that acetylcholine stimulates the muscarinic receptors on the endothelium, leading to the release of a nonprostanoid relaxing factor or EDRF. The existence of EDRF was confirmed by other studies and proved to be mainly nitric oxide or a similar chemical related compound (10,11).

B. Nitric Oxide and Its Physiology

Nitric Oxide, a small molecule composed of one atom each of nitrogen and oxygen (NO), is generated from its substrate L-arginine by a family of NO synthases. Based on their cell or organ localization, there are three distinct synthase forms identified: neuronal (nNOS), inducible (iNOS), and endothelial (eNOS).

1. NO Release

The vascular endothelial NO synthase isoform is a constitutively expressed as a 135 kDa protein. It can be activated by receptor-G protein (12,13) coupling in response to a number of stimuli (e.g. platelet release product, neurotransmitter, or circulating hormones) and is inhibited by several arginine analogous, including N^G-monomethyl-L-arginine. It can also be stimulated by physical stimuli, e.g., longitudinal sheer stress generated by blood flow. Endothelium thus responds to change in blood flow.

2. Shear-Stress-Induced release of NO by the Endothelium

Shear stress is the pressure exerted along the endothelial surface as the blood flows through the vessel. It is considered as the most important physiological stimulus for the release of NO from endothelial cells. The mechanism through which the endothelium senses the changes in shear on its surface is not fully understood. However, while responding to shear stress, endothelial cells activate the release of Ca^{2+}, which binds to calmodulin to form Ca^{2+}-calmodulin complexes, therefore, activate eNOS to synthesize NO (14,15). However, as for other agonists, shear-stress-stimulated release of NO by the endothelium involves not only calcium dependent (16), but also calcium independent mechanisms (17).

3. Cardiovascular Physiology of NO

NO has a very short half-life. It is rapidly oxidized to form mixtures of nitrite and nitrate by oxygen and oxygen free radicals. After being released from the endothelium, NO diffuses across the extracellular space into smooth muscle cells to stimulate an enhanced formation of cyclic GMP (18), an intracellular second messenger. Its elevation activates the cGMP-dependent kinase in smooth muscle cells which results in a reduction of activating calcium available for contraction (19). NO thus relaxes vascular smooth muscle to modulate the systemic vascular resistance, blood pressure (20,21) and the basal vascular tone in the coronary (22), pulmonary (12,23) and peripheral (24) circulations.

NO is not simply a vessel dilator. In addition to relaxing smooth muscle, it enhances myocardial relaxation (25) and inhibits platelet adhesion and aggregation (26-28) and smooth muscle proliferation (29) by activating guanylyl cyclase and increasing cellular cGMP. NO is also capable of reacting with NO synthase, the enzyme responsible for its own production. It has been found both *in vitro* and *in vivo* that NO attenuated NOS activity (30,31) which suggest that NO may play an important regulatory role on endothelial function through negative feedback inhibition (32).

II. Endothelial Dysfunction in Atherosclerosis

Atherosclerosis is characterized by hypertrophy of the vascular media, thickening of intima, and a core filled with cholesterol esters. Up to recent times, atherosclerosis was described as an entirely morphological entity (32). However, recent studies have demonstrated that the functional aspects of the dysfunctional endothelium are as important as its morphologic ones (34). For example, atherosclerosis is associated with impaired responsiveness to increase in blood flow (35,36) as well as to endothelium-dependent vasodilators (37,38). Endothelial dysfunction, that has been found in the early stage of atherosclerosis (6,7,39,40), plays a key role in atherogenesis. Loss of NO activity may be a marker of at least the potential for atheroma, or it may directly precede the formation of plaque (41,42). Restoration of NO activity by oral supplementation of L-arginine can induce regression of preexisting intimal lesions (43). Furthermore, all major cardiovascular risk factors have been associated with impaired endothelial function (1,7,44-47), which precedes clinically apparent vascular disease.

A. Mechanism underlying Endothelial Dysfunction in Atherosclerosis

The mechanisms underlying impairment of NO activity in atherosclerosis is insufficiently understood, and it may differ according to the specific condition.

1. Impaired NO Production

It is noteworthy that atheroma tends to occur at sites of low endothelial shear stress where NO production is low. There are several lines of evidence showing that endothelial dysfunction in atherosclerosis is due to impaired NO synthesis or release (48,49). This interpretation is supported by the evidence that infusion or oral supplementation of L-arginine, the precursor of NO, can improve endothelial function in hypercholesterolemic animals and humans (50,51). Furthermore, restoration of NO activity by oral supplementation of L-arginine can induce regression of preexisting intimal lesions (43). On the other hand, there are also studies demonstrating that L-arginine did not improve peripheral artery endothelial function in hypercholesterolemic patients and rabbits (52,53). In addition, administration of L-arginine did not restore coronary endothelial dysfunction in hypertensive patients with coronary disease (54,55). Therefore, the mechanisms responsible for the impaired endothelial function in those patients may not be NO synthesis or at least they are not related to a limited availability of L-arginine. In fact, it was found that the production of NO in atherosclerotic arteries was enhanced rather than impaired, although the amount of bio-assayable NO was reduced, when compared with controls (56), which suggests that endothelial dysfunction be related to an augmented degradation of NO.

2. Shortened NO Half-life

Several studies have found an excess production of O^{2-} in vessels from hypercholesterolemic animals and humans (57,58), which causes an augmented destruction of NO. It is true that endothelium-dependent vasodilation can be restored by superoxide dismutase (59-61) and antioxide vitamins (62) in cholesterol fed animals and in patients with diabetes mellitus (63). In addition to animal models, Vitamin C has shown beneficial effect on endothelial function in chronic smokers (64) and non-insulin-dependent diabetes mellitus (65); an antioxidant, ascorbic acid, also reversed endothelial vasomotor in patients with coronary disease (66) in humans.

Another possible mechanism for endothelial dysfunction may relate to insensitive smooth muscle response to NO. However, this mechanism is still under investigation (67-69).

III.   Detection and Quantification of Endothelial Dysfunction

While endothelial dysfunction has been clearly described using *in vitro* models and using invasive procedures *in vivo*, it is becoming increasingly clear that the most important application of this discovery would be in the primary prevention setting. Therefore, it is vital the development of a non invasive, relatively inexpensive and reliable procedure to detect and quantify endothelial dysfunction.

A. Systemic Nature of Endothelial Dysfunction

Impairment of endothelium-dependent vasodilation in the coronary arteries has been demonstrated in patients with documented atherosclerosis and/or established cardiovascular risk factors (34-37,70-72). There are also growing evidences suggesting that endothelial dysfunction is also present in patients with peripheral artery atherosclerosis (1,38,73-76). Therefore, endothelial dysfunction occurs in both the coronary and peripheral circulation during different stages of atherosclerosis (77). Thus, the systemic nature of endothelial dysfunction in atherosclerosis has prompted the development of non-invasive protocol to evaluate endothelial dysfunction in easily accessible peripheral arteries, e.g., the brachial artery.

B. Non-Invasive Assessment of Brachial Artery Vasoreactivity

Endothelial dysfunction is an early event in atherosclerosis. Many techniques have been employed to evaluate endothelium-dependent vasoreactivity in patient with atherosclerosis (1,38,78-82) with pharmacological and physiological stimuli. However, some of these procedures are invasive and cannot be performed to study asymptomatic patients nor frequently repeated over time.

Non-invasive evaluation of brachial vasoreactivity using high resolution B-mode ultrasound is currently being established to evaluate endothelial function after being first developed and introduced by Celermajer et al (78).

1. Vasodilation Test, Imaging and Data Acquisition

The subject is resting in a comfortable supine position with the arm extended in a manner allowing consistent access to the brachial artery for imaging. The brachial artery ultrasound at a location 3-7 cm above the antecubital crease (79). The image is recorded using the longitudinal view while optimizing arterial wall interfaces.

Brachial artery vasoreaction is induced by elevated NO release due to a gross increase of blood flow and shear stress produced by a sudden release of the external mechanical occlusion (i.e., inflation of a pressure cuff to suppress arm blood flow for 4.5 to 5 minutes (78-80).

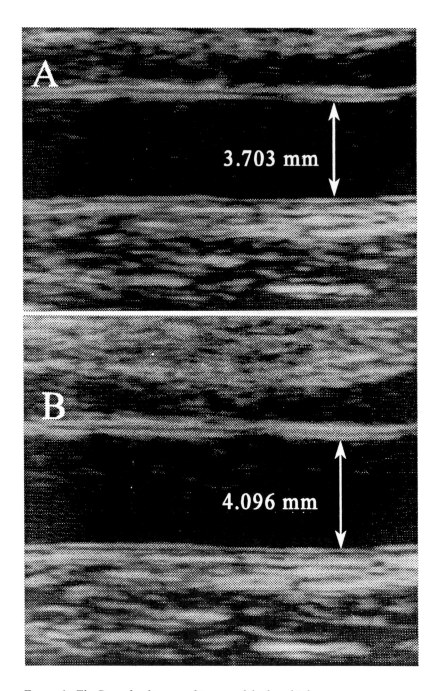

Figure 1. The B-mode ultrasound image of the brachial artery.

A. At the baseline
B. At the peak of vasoreaction

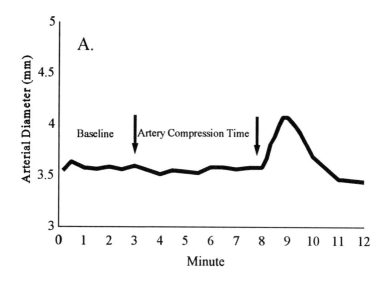

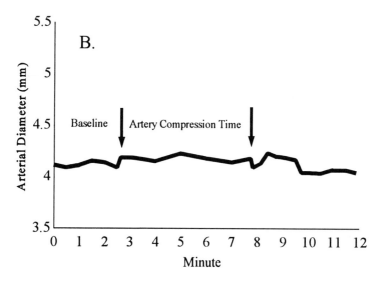

Figure 2. Brachial artery diameter (mm) as measured by B-mode ultrasound imaging (13 MHZ) during a 12 minute experiment including a 3 min baseline, 5 min proximal pressure cuff compression and 4 min reaction time.

A. 34 year old healthy female without any cardiovascular risk factors.

B. 52 year old female with hypertension.is imaged by using high-resolution B-mode

The arterial diameter is measured at the baseline and during the reactive hyperemia *(Figure 1)*. Preliminary data seem to show that there is a clear relationship between the ability of the brachial artery to dilate in response to compression and the prevalence of CHD and CVD risk factors *(Figure 2.A.B.)* It has also been observed that the peak reaction (maximum diameter change) time is around 1 minute after the pressure cuff release (79) (Figure 2.A). We have found that the peak reaction time in 50% of the subjects studied in our laboratory ranged from 46 to 71 seconds (unpublished data). Therefore, it is necessary to continuously measure the diameter for 2 minutes upon release of the occlusion to adequately evaluate the vasodilation, and to identify the peak dilation.

2. Reproducibility

A 7.0 MHZ transducer, this technique was able to identify a change in the arterial diameter of about 0.1 mm (80). The inter-observer coefficient of variation in measuring the brachial artery baseline diameter was 2.6%, and the coefficient of variation in measuring the arterial dilation in response to 5-minute external occlusion was 1.4% (78).

In duplicate scans, the coefficient of variation in evaluation of baseline diameter and vasodilation was 3.8% and 2.3%, respectively (78). In our laboratory, with a 13 MHZ transducer, the absolute differences in measuring brachial artery diameter at the baseline and the peak dilation is 0.07 mm and 0.08 mm, respectively, in repeated exams with a 0.98 correlation coefficient (Table 1). Therefore, when using a highly standardized protocol and a sensitive instrument, brachial endothelial function can be accurately and reliably evaluated by non-invasive ultrasound protocols.

Table 1. Reproducibility of B-mode Ultrasound in Measuring Flow-mediated Brachial Artery Vasoreactivity

	Mean Diameter (mm) N=9			Correlation N=9	
	1st Measure	2nd Measure	Abs. Dif.	r	p-value
Baseline	3.66±0.43	3.64±0.47	0.07	0.98	0.000
Peak Dilation	3.99±0.43	3.95±0.44	0.08	0.98	0.000

C. Arterial Reactivity and Atherogenesis

Endothelial dysfunction may become an important surrogate endpoint for detecting early signs of atherogenesis and an efficient model to test the antiatherogenic effects of medical therapy. Many investigations have been conducted to study the association of risk factor prevalence and brachial artery reactivity.

1. Aging

The prevalence of atherosclerosis increases in the elderly population. Several studies using animal models suggest a decrease in endothelial release of NO with age (81,82). Endothelium-dependent, brachial vasodilation is progressively impaired with age (72,74) in humans.

Celermajer and coworkers (83) used high resolution B-mode ultrasound to study endothelium-dependent and endothelium-independent vascular reactivity in 103 healthy men and 135 healthy women aged 15 to 72 years (38 ± 17 years). Among those, there were 36 postmenopausal women whose average age at the menopause was 51 ± 1 years and none of them was on hormone replacement therapy. In response to the increase in flow after pressure cuff deflation, there was an increase in brachial artery diameter of $7.9\pm3.9\%$ (range, -1% to 18%). In response to an endothelium independent vasodilator (i.e., glyceryl trinitrate), the arterial diameter increased by $19.4\pm5.8\%$ (range, 4% to 38%). Both flow-mediated vasodilation and glyceryl trinitrate induced vasodilation were associated with vessel size. No correlation was found between age and degree of hyperemia, or between flow-mediated dilation and hyperemia. However, age was inversely related to flow-mediated vasodilation ($r=-0.34$, $p<0.0001$) while brachial artery response to glyceryl trinitrate was preserved into old age ($r=-0.10$, $p=0.18$). This was present in healthy adults who had no other cardiovascular risk factors, such as cigarette smoking, hypertension, diabetes or hyperlipidemia. Since there was not an age-related change in the hyperemic flow response, it is not likely that the abnormality was caused by progression of atherosclerosis. Therefore, this finding suggests that aging be a determinant of endothelial dysfunction. Progressive endothelial dysfunction in the brachial artery can occur even without other cardiovascular risk factors. Therapeutic studies aimed at improving endothelial function should be studied because they may reduce the incidence of atherosclerosis that occurs with age.

2. Estrogens

An interesting pattern was also observed in the same study regarding age-related changes in arterial physiology between men and women. In men, endothelial dependent brachial vasodilation declined gradually after around 41 years of age. In women, it did not occur until the age of the menopause or around their 53rd year. However, after the change point, a steep decline of endothelium-dependent vasoreactivity took place in women due to the loss of the protective effect of estrogens. This was supported by Leiberman et al's study (84), where they measured the change in brachial artery diameter during the increase in flow induced by reactive hyperemia in nonsmoker women aged from 44 to 69 years with mild hypercholesterolemia but free of history or clinical evidence of atherosclerosis, hypertension, diabetes, cancer, liver and renal disease. Menopause occurred in these female subjects at least a year prior to the study and it was confirmed by measuring serum follicle-stimulating hormone levels. None of them were receiving hormone replacement therapy for at least 2 months before the study. After 9-week of treatment with placebo or estradiol, there was not a significant difference in endothelium-independent vasodilation between the placebo and the treatment group. However, the brachial diameter increase in response to reactive hyperemia was twice greater when patients received estrogen treatment than when they received the placebo. Blood pressure, heart rate and total cholesterol were not significantly affected. It was also observed in another study that flow-mediated, endothelium-dependent vasodilation even varied during the menstrual cycle in healthy women (85). The percentage of vasodilation in female subjects increased in the Follicular and Luteal phases when estrogen was high but decreased in the Menstrual phase when estrogen was low. These findings suggest that estrogens have a direct effect on vascular function. However, the mechanisms through which estrogens improve endothelium-dependent vasodilation have not been elucidated, but there may be a possible effect on NO production (86,87) and degradation (88).

3. Cigarette Smoking

Direct or passive cigarette smoking are established cardiovascular risk factors, and both have a significant effect in abolishing brachial endothelial function. In a study by Celermajer et al. (45), brachial artery diameter was measured using B-mode ultrasound at the baseline, during reactive hyperemia, and after sublingual glyceryl trinitrate (GTN) in healthy young adults aged 15 to 57 years. GTN caused vasodilation in both controls and smokers while flow-mediated brachial vasodilation was absent or impaired in smokers, $4.0\pm3.9\%$, (range, 0% to 17%) when compared with nonsmokers, $10\pm3.3\%$, (range, 4% to 22%). When compared current smokers with former smokers, the arterial dilation was higher in former smokers ($5.1\pm4.0\%$). Furthermore, in the smokers, brachial vasoreactivity was significantly, inversely related to a cumulative index of exposure to cigarette smoking: $6.6\pm4.0\%$ in very light smokers, $4.0\pm3.1\%$ in light smokers, $3.2\pm3.2\%$ in moderate smokers, and $2.6\pm1.2\%$ in heavy smokers.

Later, the same authors confirmed that flow-mediated brachial dilation was significantly impaired in the passive smokers and active smokers when compared to controls who had never smoked or been exposed to tobacco smoke. In addition, in the group of passive smokers, it was shown an inverse relationship between the intensity of exposure to tobacco smoke and vasodilation (89).

The above findings demonstrate a dose-dependent relationship between smoke and endothelial dysfunction in apparently healthy young adult smokers, therefore supporting a causative role for smoking in atherosclerosis. Since flow-mediated dilation was better in former smokers than in current smokers although it was impaired in both groups, it has been suggested that the effect of smoking may be reversible. The mechanism of smoking associated endothelium damage is not clear. However, it may be related to the effect of tobacco smoke on the interaction between platelets and the vessel wall (90) or on oxidation products (91) or plasma lipid (92-94).

4. Hypercholesterolemia and Risk Factor Interaction

Endothelium-dependent vasodilation in coronary and peripheral arteries is blunted in hypercholesterolemic patients (1,44,70,71,95). Sorensen et al. (44) evaluated vasodilation in 30 familial hypercholesterolemic (FH) children, aged 7 to 17, and compared it with that of 30 healthy age and sex matched controls in the superficial femoral artery. In children with FH, total cholesterol was 240-696 mg/dl, and the flow-mediated vasodilation was significantly reduced when compared with their controls ($1.2\pm0.4\%$ verses $7.5\pm0.7\%$, $p<0.0001$). Besides endothelium-dependent vasodilation, glyceryl trinitrate induced endothelium-independent dilation was less in FH children as well ($p=0.023$). These findings show that hypercholesterolemia impairs arterial function by damaging not only the endothelium, but also smooth muscles, and that this process can begin as early as in the first decade of life. Cholesterol lowering therapy should be considered for those children although there is still some concern about the safety of this therapeutic strategy and its effects on their growth and development.

Other studies have investigated the effects of isolated cardiovascular risk factors. The interaction between risk factors and endothelial dysfunction was studied by Celermajer et al. (45), including high cholesterol, current or former smoking habit, family history, male gender, and age>50 years. In the 500 clinically well characterized male and female aged 5 to 73 years subjects (45), cholesterol level, smoking, blood pressure, family history, age and gender were all significantly associated to endothelial dysfunction. The risk factor score was independently related to brachial endothelium-dependent vasodilation even when its constituents were represented in the multivariate model, and adding the score to the model did not change the level of significance of the other risk factors, suggesting an interaction between all or some of the risk factors. This was supported by the evidence that the impact of cholesterol level was lost in heavy smokers and low cholesterol level could modify the adverse effect of smoking in moderate smokers.

5. Hypertension

Hypertension is associated with an increased risk of cardiovascular complications and coronary disease. It has been found that patients with essential hypertension have a defect in NO release both under basal conditions and during activation of the endothelium (4,54,73,96). A study with 13 essential hypertensive subjects and 13 well-matched controls documented that brachial endothelium-dependent vasodilation diminished in the hypertensive group ($13.1\pm1.6\%$ vs. $18.5\pm1.9\%$, $p<0.05$) (97). Since all the subjects were nonsmokers, free of diabetes mellitus, hyperlipidemia and atherosclerosis, it was unlikely that the endothelial function was affected by other risk factors or medication. The role of endothelial dysfunction, a secondary phenomenon or a primary etiologic role, in hypertension is not well understood. Recent studies suggest that the endothelial dysfunction be the primary mechanism in the development of hypertension and atherosclerosis in these patients (73,98).

6. Diabetes Mellitus

Diabetic patients are susceptible to increased morbidity and mortality due to vascular complications such as hypertension and atherosclerosis. Although this is still controversial (67,99-101), there are studies showing impaired endothelium-dependent vasodilation in both type 1 and type 2 diabetes mellitus (67,101,102). The mechanism by which diabetes contributes to endothelial dysfunction is unclear. It was suggested that the impaired vasoreactivity was related only to hyperinsulinemia, but in at least one study, this was not related to the duration of the disease (101). Other studies have suggested that disease duration and LDL-C were the affecting parameters (102) in type 1 diabetes. However, since in the latter study, systolic blood pressure and cholesterol levels were significantly higher in the diabetic group, it is possible that those factors, instead of diabetes *per se*, could have accounted for endothelial dysfunction or in alternative that there were interactions between these factors with the endothelium. In addition, while some studies suggested that hyperglycemia was the initiating insult (103,104), there were data showing no correlation between endothelial dysfunction and glucose concentration (101). Furthermore, by evaluating endothelium-dependent brachial vasodilation in type 1 diabetes with normoalbuminuria, it was found that the endothelial function in diabetic subjects was comparable with that in their controls (100). Therefore, hyperglycemia *per se* may be necessary but not sufficient to cause endothelial dysfunction in type 1 diabetes.

Since case control studies have demonstrated the association between endothelial dysfunction and risk factors and atherosclerosis, long-term follow-up studies would be required to determine whether subjects with abnormal endothelium-dependent vasodilation are associated with subsequent atherosclerotic disease in later life.

7. Evaluation of Therapeutic Effects

Brachial vasoreactivity can also be used as a surrogate to evaluate the effect of antiatherosclerotic therapies. It has been shown that brachial endothelial dysfunction can be improved by dietary supplementation of L-arginine, the NO substrate (51). Clarkson et al assessed flow-mediated brachial vasoreactivity in 27 hypercholesterolemic subjects with known endothelial dysfunction. After 4 weeks oral administration of L-arginine, there was a significant raise in plasma arginine and improvement of endothelium-dependent brachial vasodilation while there was no change in endothelium-independent vasodilation and lipid profiles. This could imply that L-arginine has therapeutic application. The mechanism under which L-arginine may improve endothelial function could be through the increase in NO production to balance the elevated NO inactivation by oxidized LDL-cholesterol and/or Lp(a).

In a group of 7 healthy, normocholesterolemic (LDL<160 mg/dl) middle-aged men, after administration of simvastatin, flow-mediated brachial vasoreactivity increased from baseline's 5.0% to 10.5%, 13.3%, and 15.7% with the lowering of LDL cholesterol (105). The vasodilation fell to 4.4±1.3% when cholesterol went back to baseline level 12 weeks after discontinuation the therapy (Table 2). Interestingly, the vasodilation changed with time but not perfectly with the level of LDL. Since this study did not test the significance of the differences in vasodilation and LDL levels between those weeks, it is hard to determine if lowering LDL *per se* was the only factor affecting the endothelial function. It was also possible that one or more lipid fractions that are important in endothelial function were altered. Further studies are needed to resolve this issue.

In addition, 2 hours after oral administration of ascorbic acid, an antioxidant, in 46 patients with coronary artery disease, their brachial endothelium-dependent dilation improved significantly from 6.3±1.1% to 9.5±1.2% while there was no change in the placebo group (4.4±1.1% to 3.4±1.2%)(66). When only subjects with impaired vasodilation (<5%), 13 from ascorbate group and 10 from the placebo group, were compared, ascorbic acid produced a marked increase in vasodilation (from 2.0±0.6% to 9.7±2.0%) while there was no significant change in the placebo group (1.1±0.9% to 1.7±1.5%).

Table 2. *LDL Cholesterol and Brachial Artery Vasodilation at Baseline, During Simvastatin Therapy, and After Therapy. Values expressed as Mean±SD. (Adapted from reference 105).*

	Baseline	On Simvastatin			After Simvastatin	
		2 week	4 week	12 week	4 week	12 week
LDL (mg/dL)	133±14	88±15	95±17	80±13	137±27	120±10
Vasodilation (%)	5.0±3.6	10.5±5.6	13.3±4.3	15.7±4.9	8.8±2.9	4.4±1.3

Due to the small sample size and short duration of the investigation, it is difficult to definitively prove whether these agents have long-term beneficial effect on endothelial function and the exact mechanism by which the agents affect vascular function and impact on the atherogenic process. Therefore, prospective studies with larger population are required. Since therapeutic agents affect endothelial function quickly, the evaluation of endothelium-dependent vasodilation can be useful in determining the therapeutic value of agents.

IV. Summary

Endothelial dysfunction is an early event in atherosclerosis. One manifestation of endothelial dysfunction is altered vasoreactivity. Due to its systemic nature, detecting endothelial dysfunction in an easily accessing peripheral artery may be a marker of the early stage of atherosclerosis. Brachial artery vasoreactivity has been proved to be closely related with coronary artery disease, peripheral artery disease, and several cardiovascular risk factors and can be improved by medical interventions. The non-invasive ultrasound assessment of brachial flow-mediated vasodilation is a useful surrogate for detecting endothelial function. This method is ideal for identifying asymptomatic patient at risk for atherosclerosis and assessing the effect of medication aimed at restoring endothelial function and altering or averting atherosclerosis progression.

References:

1. Creager MA, Cooke JP, Mendelsohn ME, et al: Impaired Vasodilation of Forearm Resistance Vessels in Hypercholesterolemic Humans. J Clin Invest 1990; 86:228-234.
2. Zeiher AM, Drexler HD, Wollschlager H, et al: Modulation of Coronary Vasomotor Tone in Humans: Progressive Endothelial Dysfunction with Different Early Stages of Coronary Atherosclerosis. Circulation 1991; 83:391-401.
3. Galle J, Busse R, Bassenge E: Hypercholesterolemia and Atherosclerosis Change Vascular Reactivity in Rabbits by Different Mechanisms. Arterioscler and Thromb 1991; 11:1712-1718.
4. Panza JA, Quyyumi AA, Brush JE, et al: Abnormal Endothelium-dependent Vascular Relaxation in Patients with Essential Hypertension. N Engl J Med 1990; 323:22-27.
5. Quyyumi AA, Cannon R, Panza JA, et al: Endothelial Dysfunction in Patients with Chest Pain and Normal Coronary Arteries. Circulation 1992; 86:1864-1871.
6. Reddy KG, Nair N, Sheehan HM, et al: Evidence That Selective Endothelial Dysfunction May Occur in the Absences of Angiographic or Ultrasound Atherosclerosis in Patients With Risk Factors for Atherosclerosis. J Am Coll Cardiol 1994; 23:833-843.
7. Nishimura RA, Lerman A, Chesebro JH, et al: Epicardial Vasomotor Response to Acetylcholine Are not Predicted by Coronary Atherosclerosis As Assessed by Intracoronary Ultrasound. J Am Coll Cardiol 1995; 26:41-49.
8. Badimon L, Badimon JJ, Penny W, et al: Endothelium and Atherosclerosis. J Hypertension 1992; 10(suppl 2):S43-S50.
9. Furchgott RF, Zawadzki JV: The obligatory role of endothelial cells in the relaxation of arterial smooth muscle by acetylcholine. Nature 1980; 288:373-6.

10. Ignarro LJ, Byrns, RC, Buga GM, et al: Endothelium-deride relaxing factor from pulmonary artery and vein possesses pharmacologic and chemical properties identical to those of nitric oxide radical. Circ Res 1987; 61:886-879

11. Feelisch M, te Poel M, Zamora R, et al: Understanding the controversy over the identity of EDRF. Nature 1994; 368:62-65.

12. Birnbaumer L: G-proteins in signal transduction. Annu Rev Pharmacol Toxicol 1990; 30:675-705.

13. Flavahan NA: G-proteins and Endothelial Responses. Blood Vessels 1990; 27:218-29.

14. Rubanyi GM, Romero JC, Vanhoutte PM: Flow-induced Release of Endothelium-derived relaxing Factor. Am J Physiol 1986; 250:H1145-9.

15. Pohl U, Holtz J, Busse R, et al: Critical Role of Endothelium in the Vasodilator Response to Increased Flow in vivo. Hypertension 1986; 8:37-44.

16. Kuchan MJ, Frangos JA: Role of Calcium and Calmodulin in Flow-induced Nitric Oxide production in Endothelial Cells. Am J Physiol 1994; 266:C628-36.

17. Ziegelstein RC, Cheng L, Capogrossi MC: Flow-Dependent Cytosolic Acidification of Vascular Endothelial Cells. Science 1992; 258:656-9.

18. Rapoport RM, Murad F: Agonist-induced Endothelium-Dependent relaxation in Rat Thoracic Aorta may be mediated through cguanosine monophosphate. Cir Res 1983; 52:352-7.

19. Lincoln TM: Cyclic GMP and Mechanisms of Vasodilation. Pharmacolo Ther 1989; 41:479-502.

20. Ress DD, Palmer RMJ, Moncada S: Role of Endothelium-Derived Nitric Oxide in the Regulation of Blood Pressure. Proc Natl Acad Sci USA 1989; 86;3375-3378.

21. Stamler JS, Loh E, Roddy M, et al: Nitric Oxide Regulates Basal Systemic and Pulmonary Vascular Resistance in Healthy Humans. Circulation 1994; 89:2.35-2040.

22. Drexler H, Zeiher AM, Wollschlager R, et al: Flow dependent coronary artery dilation in Humans. Circulation 1989; 80:466-74.

23. Cooper CJ, Landzberg MJ, Anderson TJ, et al: Role of Nitric Oxide in the Local Regulation of Pulmonary Vascular Resistance in Humans. Circulation 1996; 93:266-271.

24. Vallance P, Collier J, Moncada S: Effects of Endothelium-derived Nitric Oxide on Peripheral Arteriolar Tone in Man. Lancet 1989; 2:997-1000.

25. Grocott-Mason R, Anning P, Evans H, et al: Modulation of Left Ventricular Relaxation in Isolated Ejecting Heart by Endogenous Nitric Oxide. Am J Physiol 1994; 267:H1804-13.

26. Radomski MW, Palmer RMJ, Moncada S: Endogenous Nitric Oxide Inhibits Human Platelet Adhesion to the Vascular Endothelium. Lancet 1987; 2:1057-1058.

27. de Graaf J, Banga JD, Moncada S, et al: Nitric Oxide Functions as an Inhibitor of Platelet Adhesion Under Flow Conditions. Circulation 1992; 85:2284-2290.

28. Yan Z, Yokota T, Zhang W, et al: Expression of Inducible Nitric Oxide Synthase Inhibits Platelet Adhesion and Restores Blood Flow in the Injured Artery. Circ Res 1996; 79:38-44.

29. Mooradian DL, Hutsell TC, and Keefer LK: Nitric Oxide (NO. Donor Molecules: Effect of NO Release Rate on Vascular Smooth Muscle Cell Proliferation In Vitro. J Cardiovasc Pharmacol 1995; 25:674-678.

30. Rengasamy A and Johns RA: Regulation of Nitric Oxide Synthase by Nitric Oxide. Mol Pharmacol 1993; 44:124-128.

31. Ravichandran LV, Johns RA, and Rengasamy A: Direct and Reversible Inhibition of Endothelial Nitric Oxide Synthase by Nitric Oxide. Am J Physiol 1995; 268:H2216-2223.

32. Buga GM, Griscavage JM, Rogers NE, et al: Negative Feedback Regulation of Endothelial Cell Function by Nitric Oxide. Circ Res 1993; 73:808-812.

33. Ross R: The Pathogenesis of Atherosclerosis. N Engl J Med 1986; 314:488-500.

34. Forstermann U, Mugge A, Alheid U, et al: Selective Attenuation of Endothelium-Derived Vasodilation in Atherosclerotic Human Coronary Arteries. Circ Res 1988; 62:185-190.

35. Nabel EG, Selwyn AP, Ganz P: Large Coronary Arteries in Humans Are Responsive to Changing Blood Flow: An Endothelium-Dependent Mechanism that Fails in Patients with Atherosclerosis. J Am Coll Cardiol 1990; 16:349-356.

36. Cox DA, Vita JA, Treasure CB, et al: Atherosclerosis Impairs Flow-Mediated Dilation of Coronary Arteries in Humans. Circulation 1989; 80:458-465.

37. Zeiher AM, Drexler H, Wollschlager H, et al: Modulation of Coronary Vasomotor Tone in Humans: Progressive Endothelial dysfunction with different Early Stage of Coronary Atherosclerosis. Circulation 1991; 83:391-401.

38. Liao JK, Bettmann MA, Sandor T, et al: Differential Impairment of Vasodilator Responsiveness of Peripheral Resistance and Conduit Vessels in Humans With Atherosclerosis. Circ Res 1991; 68:1027-1034.

39. Davis SF, Yeung AC, Meredith IT, et al: Early Endothelial Dysfunction Predicts the Development of Transplant Coronary Artery Disease at 1 Year Posttransplant. Circulation 1996; 93:457-462.

40. Zeiher AM, Drexler H, Wollschlager H, et al: Modulation of Coronary Vasomotor Tone in Humans: Progressive Endothelial Dysfunction with Different Early Stages of Coronary Atherosclerosis. Circulation 1991; 83:391-40.

41. Cooke JP, Tsao PS: Is NO an Endogenous Antiatherogenic Molecule. Arterioscler Throm 1994; 14:653-655

42. Luscher TF: The Endothelium As a Target and Mediator of Cardiovascular Disease. Eur j Clin Invest 1993; 23:670-685.

43. Candipan RC, Wang B, Buitrago R, et al: Regression of Progression. Dependency on Vascular Nitric Oxide. Arterioscler Thromb and Biol 1996; 16:44-50.

44. Sorensen KE, Celermajer DS, Georggakopoulos D, et al: Impairment of Endothelium-Dependent Dilation Is an Early Event in Children with Familial Hypercholesterolemia and Is Related to the Lipoprotein (a) Level. J Clin Invest 1994; 93:50-55.

45. Celermajer DS, Sorensen KE, Bull C, et al: Endothelium-Dependent Dilation in the Systemic Arteries of Asymptomatic Subjects Relates to Coronary Risk Factors and Their Interaction. J Am Coll Cardiol 1994; 24:1468-1474.

46. Celermajer DS, Sorensen KE, Gooch VM, et al: Non-Invasive Detection of Endothelial Dysfunction in Children and Adults at Risk of Atherosclerosis. Lancet 1992; 340:1111-1115.

47. Iiyama K, Naagano M, Yo Y, et al: Impaired Endothelial Function With Essential Hypertension Assessed by Ultrasonography. Am Heart J 1996; 132:779-782.

48. Lefer AM, Ma XL: Decreased Basal Nitric Oxide Release in Hypercholesterolemia Increases Neutrophil Adherence to Coronary Artery Endothelium. Arterioscler Thromb 1993; 13:771-776.

49. Chester AH, O'Neil GS, Moncada S, et al: Low Basal and Stimulated Release of Nitric Oxide in Atherosclerotic Epicardial Coronary Arteries. Lancet 1990; 336:897-900.

50. Girerd XJ, Hirsch AT, Cooke JP, et al: L-Arginine Augments Endothelium-Dependent Vasodilation in Cholesterol-Fed Rabbits. Circ Res 1990 ; 67:1301-1308.

51. Clarkson P, Adams MR, Powe AJ, et al: Oral L-Arginine Improves Endothelium-Dependent Dilation in Hypercholesterolemic Young Adults. J Clin Invest 1996; 97:1989-1994.

52. Wennmalm A, Edlund A, Granstrom EF, et al: Acute Supplementation with the Nitric Oxide Precursor L-Arginine Does not Improve Cardiovascular Performance in Patients with Hypercholesterolemia. Atherosclerosis 1995; 118:223-231.

53. Jeremy RW, McCarron H, Sullivan D: Effects of Dietary L-Arginine on Atherosclerosis and Endothelium-dependent Vasodilation in the Hypercholesterolemic Rabbit. Response According to Treatment Duration, Anatomic Site, and Sex. Circulation 1996; 94:498-506.

54. Panza JA, Casino PR, Badar DM, et al: Effect of Increased Availability of Endothelium-derived Nitric Oxide Precursor on Endothelium-dependent Vascular Relaxation in Normal Subjects and in Patients with Essential Hypertension. Circulation 1993; 87:1475-1481.

55. Hirooka Y, Egashira K, Imaizumi T, et al: Effect of L-Arginine on Acetylcholine-Induced Endothelium-Dependent Vasodilation Differs Between the Coronary and Forearm Vasculars in Humans. J Am Coll Cardiol 1994; 24:948-955.

56. Minor RL Jr, Myers PR, Guerra R Jr, et al: Diet-Induced Atherosclerosis Increases the Release of Nitrogen Oxides from Rabbit Aorta. J Clin Invest 1990; 86:2109-2116.

57. Ohara Y, Peterson TE, Harrison DG: Hypercholesterolemia Increases Endothelial Superoxide Anion Production. J Clin Invest 1993; 91:2546-2551.

58. Mugge A, Brandes RP, Boger RH, et al: Vascular Release of Superoxide Radicals is Enhanced in hypercholesterolemic Rabbits. J Cardiovasc Pharmacol 1994; 24:994-998.

59. Tesfamariam B, Cohen RA: Free Radical Mediate Endothelial Cell Dysfunction Caused by Elevated Glucose. Am J Physiol 1992; 90:727-732.

60. Mugge A, Elwell JH, Peterson TE, et al: Chronic Treatment with Polyethylene-Glycolated Superoxide Dismutase Partially Restores Endothelium-Dependent Vascular Relaxations in Cholesterol-Fed Rabbits. Circ Res 1991; 69:1293-1300.

61. Hattori Y, Kawaski H, Abe K, et al: Superoxide Dismutase Recovers Altered Endothelium-Dependent Relaxation in Diabetic Rat Aorta. Am J Physiol 1991; 261:H1086-H1094.

62. Keaney JFJ, Gaziiano JM, Xu Z, et al: Dietary Antioxidants Preserve Endothelium-Dependent Vessel Relaxation in Cholesterol-Fed Rabbits. Proc Natl Acad Sci USA, 1993; 90:11880-11884.

63. Hattori Y, Kawaski H, Abe K, et al: Superoxide Dismutase Recovers Altered Endothelium-Dependent Relaxation in Diabetic Rat Aorta. Am J Physiol 1991; 261:H1086-H1094.

64. Heitzer T, Just H, Munzel T: Antioxidant Vitamin C Improves Endothelial Dysfunction in Chronic Smokers. Circulation 1996; V4:6-9.

65. Ting HH, Timimi FK, Boles KS, et al: Vitamin C Improves Endothelium-Dependent Vasodilation in Patients with Non-Insulin-Dependent Diabetes Mellitus. J Clin Invest 1996; 97:22-28.

66. Levine GN, Frei B, Koulouris SN, et al: Ascorbic Acid Reverses Endothelial Vasomotor Dysfunction in Patients With Coronary Artery Disease. Circulation 1996; 93:1107-1113.
67. Williams SB, Cusco JA, Roddy M, et al: Impaired Nitric Oxide-Mediated Vasodilation in Patients With Non-Insulin-Dependent Diabetes Mellitus. J Am Cardiol 1996; 27:567-574.
68. Gupta S, Sussman I, McArthur CS, et al: Endothelium-Dependent Inhibition of NA+-K+ ATPase Activity in Rabbit Aorta by Hyperglycemia: Possible Role of Endothelium-Derived Nitric Oxide. J Clin Invest 1992; 90:727-732.
69. Weisbrod RM, Griswold MC, Du Y, et al: Reduced Responsiveness of Hypercholesterolemic Rabbit Aortic Smooth Muscle Cells to Nitric Oxide. Arterioscler Thromb Vasc Biol 1997; 17:394-402.
70. Vita JA, Treasure CB, Nabel EG, et al: Coronary Vasomotor Response to Acetylcholine Relates to Risk Factors for Coronary Artery Disease. Circulation 1990; 81:491-497.
71. Egashira K, Inou T, Hirooka Y, et al: Impaired Coronary Artery Blood Flow Response to Acetylcholine in Patients With Coronary Risk Factors and Proximal Atherosclerotic Lesions. J Clin Invest 1993; 91:29-37.
72. Egashira K, Inou T, Hirooka Y, et al: Effects of Age on Endothelium-Dependent Vasodilation of Coronary Resistance Artery by Acetylcholine in Humans. Circulation 1993; 88:77-81.
73. Taddei S, Virdis A, Mattei P, et al: Defective L-Arginine-Nitric Oxide Pathway in Offspring of Essential Hypertensive Patients. Circulation 1996; 94:1298-1303.
74. Gerhard M, Roddy M, Creager SJ, et al: Aging Progressively Impairs Endothelium-Dependent Vasodilation in Forearm Resistance Vessels of Humans. Hypertension 1996; 27:849-853.
75. Johnstone MT, Creager SJ, Scales KM, et al: Impaired Endothelium-Dependent Vasodilation in Patients With Insulin-Dependent Diabetes Mellitus. Circulation 1993; 88:2510-2516.
76. Harris LM, Faggioli GL, Shah R, et al: Vascular Reactivity in Patients With Peripheral Vascular Disease. Am J Cardiol 1995; 76:207-212.
77. Anderson TJ, Uehata A, Gerhard MD, et al: Close relationship of Endothelial Function in the Human Coronary and Peripheral Circulations. J Am Coll Cardiol 1995; 26:1235-1241.
78. Celermajer DS, Sorensen KE, Gooch VM, et al: Non-invasive Detection of Endothelial Dysfunction in Children and Adults at Risk of Atherosclerosis. Lancet 1992; 340:1111-1115.
79. Corretti MA, Plotnick GD, Vogel RA, et al: Technical Aspects of Evaluating of Brachial Artery Vasodilation Using High-Frequency Ultrasound. Am J Physiol 1995; 37:H1397-H1404.
80. Sorensen KE, Clermajer DS, Spiegelhalter DJ, et al: Non-invasive Measurement of Human Endothelium Dependent Arterial Responses: Accuracy and Reproducibility. Br Heart J 1995; 74:247-253.
81. Mayhan WG, Faraci FM, Baumbach GL, et al: Effect of Aging on Response of Cerebral Arterioles. Am J physiol 1990; 258:H1138-H1143.
82. Luscher TF, Tanner FC, Dohi Y: Age, Hypertension, and Hypercholesterolemia Alter Endothelium-Dependent Vascular Regulation. Pharmacol Toxicol 1992; 70:s32-s39.
83. Celermajer DS, Sorensen KE, Spiegelhalter DJ, et al: Aging Is Associated With Endothelial Dysfunction in Healthy Men Years Before the Age-Related Decline in Women. J Am Coll Cardiol 1994; 24:471-476.
84. Leiberman EH, Gerhard MD, Uehata A, et al: Estrogen Improves Endothelium-Dependent, Flow-Mediated Vasodilatoin in Postmenopausal Women. Ann Intern Med 1994; 121:936-941.
85. Hashimoto M, Akishita M, Eto M, et al: Modulation of Endothelium-Dependent Flow-Mediated Dilatation of the Brachial Artery By Sex and Menstrual Cycle. Circulation 1995; 92:3431-3435.
86. Gillian DM, Quyyumi AA, Cannon RO: Effects of Physiological Levels of Estrogen On Coronary Vasomotor Function in Postmenopausal Women. Circulation 1994; 89:2545-2551.
87. Weiner CP, Lizasoain I, Baylis SA, et al: Induction of Calcium-Dependent Nitric Oxide Synthases by Sex Hormones. Proc Natl Acad Sci USA 1994; 91:5212-5216.
88. Keaney JF Jr, Shwaery GT, Xu A, et al: 17-b-estradiol preserves endothelial vasodilator function ans Limits Low-density Lipoprotein Oxidation in Hypercholesterolemic Swine. Circulation 1994; 89:2251-2259.
89. Celermajer DS, Adams MR, Clarkson P, et al: Passive Smoking and Impaired Endothelium-Dependent Arterial Dilation in Healthy Young Adults. N Engl J Med 1996; 334:150-154.
90. Burghuber OC, Punzengruber C, Sinzinger H, et al: Platelet Sensitivity to Prostacyclin in Smokers and Non-smokers. Chest 1986; 90:34-8.
91. Duthie GG, Arthur JR, James WP: Effects of Smoking and vitamin E on Blood Antioxidant Status. Am J Clin Nutr 1991; 53(suppl):1061S-1063S.
92. Moskowitz WB, Mosteller M, Schieken RM, et al: Lipoprotein and Oxygen Transport Alterations in Passive Smoking Preadolescent Children. Circulation 1990; 81:586-592.
93. Higman DJ, Strachan AMJ, Buttery L, et al: Smoking Impairs the Activity of Endothelial Nitric Oxide Synthase in Saphenous Vein. Arterioscler Thromb Vasc Biol 1996;1 6:546-552.
94. Princen HMG, van Poppel G, Vogelezang C, et al: Supplementation with Vitamin E But Not b-Carotene in Vivo Protects Low Density Lipoprotein From Lipid Peroxidation in Vitro Effect of Cigarette Smoking. Arterioscler Thromb 1992; 12:554-562.

95. Casion PR, Kilcoyne CM, Quyyumi AA, et al: The Role of Nitric Oxide in Endothelium-dependent Vasodilation of Hypercholesterolemic Patients. Circulation 1993; 88:2541-2547.
96. Taddei S, Virdis A, Mattei P, et al: Vasodilation to Acetylcholine in Primary and Secondary Forms of Human Hypertension. Hypertension 1993; 21:929-933.
97. Iiyama K, Nagano M, Yo Y, et a: Impaired Endothelial Function with Essential Hypertension Assessed by Ultrasonography. Am Hear J 1996; 132:77-82.
98. Taddei S, Virdis A, Mattei P, et al: Endothelium-Dependent Forearm Vasodilation is Reduced in Normotensive Subjects with a Family History of Hypertension. J Cardiovsc Pharmacol 1992; 20(suppl 7):S179-S195.
99. Bohlen HG and Lash JM: Endothelial-Dependent Vasodilation Is Preserved in Non-Insulin-Dependent Zucker Fatty Diabetic Rats. Am J Physiol 1995; 268:H2366-H2374
100. Lambert J, Aarsen M, Donker Ab JM, et al: Endothelium-Dependent and -Independent Vasodilation of Large Arteries in Normoalbuminuric Insulin-Dependent Diabetes Mellitus. Arterioscler Thromb Vasc Biol 1996; 16:705-711.
101. Johnstone MT, Creager SJ, Scales KM, et al: Impaired Endothelium-Dependent Vasodilation in Patients With Insulin-Dependent Diabetes Mellitus. Circulation 1993; 88:2510-2516.
102. Clarkson P, Celermajer DS, Donald AE, et al: Impaired Vascular Reactivity in Insulin-Dependent Diabetes Mellitus Is Related to Disease Duration and Low Density Lipoprotein Cholesterol Levels. J Am Coll Cardiol 1996; 28:573-579.
103. Makimattila S, Virkamaki A, Groop PH, et al: Chronic Hyperglycemia Impairs Endothelial Function and Insulin Sensitivity Via Different Mechanisms in Insulin-Dependent Diabetes Mellitus. Circulation 1996; 94:1276-1282.
104. Poston L, Taylor PD: Endothelium Mediated Vascular Function in Insulin-Dependent Diabetes Mellitus. Clin Sci 1995; 88:245-255.
105. Vogel RA, Corretti MC, Plotnick GD: Changes in Flow-Mediated Brachial Artery Vasoactivity With Lowering of Desirable Cholesterol Levels in Healthy Middle-Aged Men. Am J Cardiol 1996; 77:37-40.

QUANTITATIVE B-MODE ULTRASOUND IMAGING IN OBSERVATIONAL STUDIES

Michiel L. Bots, M.D., Ph.D. and Diederick E. Grobbee, M.D., Ph.D.

Utrecht University Medical School
Utrecht, The Netherlands

Contents

I. INTRODUCTION

Cardiovascular disease constitutes an important cause of morbidity and mortality in industrialized countries. This applies particularly to the elderly, in which they represent by far the leading cause of death and a major source of chronic impairment (1). The past decades have led to a better understanding of the etiology and pathogenesis of atherosclerosis and its clinical sequelae. Several observational studies have identified risk factors such as elevated serum cholesterol, high blood pressure, smoking and elevated levels of fibrinogen. These factors promote atherogenesis and significantly increase the risk of cardiovascular disease.

The mechanisms which cause atherosclerosis have not been sufficiently elucidated yet. Furthermore, knowledge on factors which may trigger clinical events to occur in the presence or absence of atherosclerotic abnormalities is limited (2). Thus, the question why some people suffer from a cardiovascular event whereas others may be spared from symptomatic cardiovascular disease remains unanswered. This is particularly important for subjects of older age in whom atherosclerosis is highly prevalent, though its severity varies.

Evidence for the presence of 'trigger' factors may be found in the pattern of occurrence of atherosclerotic cardiovascular disease. For angina pectoris, myocardial infarction and sudden cardiac death, circadian variation in occurrence has been documented (3,4). Circadian variation in 'trigger' factors may be the likely underlying mechanism to this phenomenon, rather than the circadian expression of atherosclerosis severity (Figure 1). For hemostatic and fibrinolytic factors circadian rhythms have been described (5). In addition, in the Physicians Health Study a circadian variation of incidence of myocardial infarction could not be demonstrated in subjects that were on aspirin treatment, yet was found for those on placebo (6). These results indicate that factors involved in clotting mechanisms may constitute 'trigger' factors for symptomatic disease in subjects with atherosclerotic vascular changes. Further research in this area is needed, in particular to study which factors may cause events to occur in the absence or presence of atherosclerosis. This notion stresses the importance of the use of non-invasive techniques to validly detect early and advanced stages of atherosclerosis in large samples of populations. The main goal for non-invasive observational studies is to gain knowledge of the mechanisms that lead to the occurrence of cardiovascular disease and its relation with prevalence and progression of atherosclerosis.

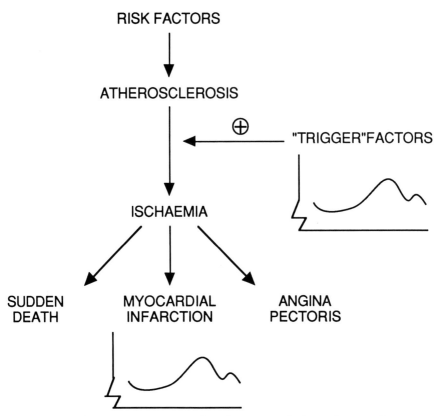

Figure 1. Schematic presentation of mechanisms underlying the circadian variation in 'trigger' factors and the role of atherosclerosis herein.

II. NON-INVASIVE ASSESSMENT OF ATHEROSCLEROSIS

Several non-invasive approaches can be used to study atherosclerosis in observational studies. The value of the ankle-arm index measurement in atherosclerosis research has been recognized for decades (7). This method provides information on the extent of atherosclerosis of arteries of the lower extremities based on flow disturbances. Direct information on vessel wall abnormalities can, however, not be obtained. In addition, the ankle-arm index is less suitable for detection of small abnormalities since those do not lead to detectable flow disturbances. Yet, the ankle-arm index has proven to be a strong predictor of cardiovascular disease and all-cause mortality (7).

A method which has not received very much attention is the indirect assessment of atherosclerosis in the abdominal aorta. This can be accomplished by measuring the presence and extent of aortic calcifications using a plain X-ray of the lumbar spine region (8). Assessment of aortic calcifications is a valid and specific tool to gain information on advanced aortic atherosclerotic lesions. Presence of aortic calcifications has been shown to be a strong predictor of cardiovascular disease and mortality (9). Furthermore, the same technique has been used to determine changes over time in atherosclerosis of the aorta (10). However, early vessel wall abnormalities cannot be detected.

The use of ultrafast computer tomography and magnetic resonance imaging as non-invasive techniques to address coronary atherosclerosis has been reported recently, and holds promising possibilities for the future (11-3). However the presently high cost and time constraint would probably hold these techniques off the observational studies as for now.

In recent years, high resolution B-mode ultrasonography has been used extensively to study the process of atherosclerosis (14-8). High resolution B-mode ultrasonography enables us to study vessel wall characteristics of superficial arteries in an effective and accurate way. This technique facilitates the evaluation of the lumen diameter, the intima-media thickness and the presence and extent of plaques and can be applied in both the carotid artery and the femoral artery (19). The remainder of the article will focus on carotid intima-media thickness measurements since most of the currently available experience is based on this measurement.

III. DESCRIPTION OF MAJOR OBSERVATIONAL STUDIES

At present, at least four major population-based observational studies are ongoing using carotid ultrasound to study the process of atherosclerosis (14-6,20). In these studies the participants were randomly sampled from the general population. There is a considerable number of other population-based studies currently going on among smaller groups of participants (21-3). The general characteristics of several studies are described in Table 1. The fourth Tromso survey has just finished to perform the baseline data collection including ultrasound measurements (Bonaa K, personal communication).

Table 1.   General characteristics of population-based observational studies using intima-media thickness measurements

Study (Ref.)	Baseline collection	Men (N.)	Women (N.)	Age range	Outcome variable
ARIC (14)	1988-1990	6335	7770	45-64	CCA-BIF-ICA $\bar{x}$ maximum IMT
Bruneck (21)	1990	460	449	40-79	plaque score
CHS (15)	1989-1990	2255	2946	65-102	CCA-BIF-ICA $\bar{x}$ maximum IMT
France (23)	1988-1989	none	517	45-54	plaques and IMT
Italy (22)	1989-1990	630	718	18-99	plaque score
KIHD (16)	1987-1989	1252	none	40,48, 54,60	CCA-BIF $\bar{x}$ maximum IMT
RS (20)	1990-1993	3105	4878	55-106	CCA-BIF $\bar{x}$ of $\bar{x}$ IMT
Tromso	1994-1995	3300	3500	25-99	CCA-BIF $\bar{x}$ maximum IMT or $\bar{x}$ of $\bar{x}$ IMT

IMT = intima-media thickness; CCA = common carotid artery; BIF = carotid bifurcation; ICA = internal carotid artery; $\bar{x}$ = mean

A. Assessment of Intima-Media Thickness

All studies listed in Table 1 use the longitudinal image of the carotid artery to perform the intima-media thickness measurements. On a longitudinal 2-dimensional ultrasound image of the carotid artery, the near and far wall of the carotid artery are displayed as two bright white lines separated by a hypo-echogenic space (Figure 2).

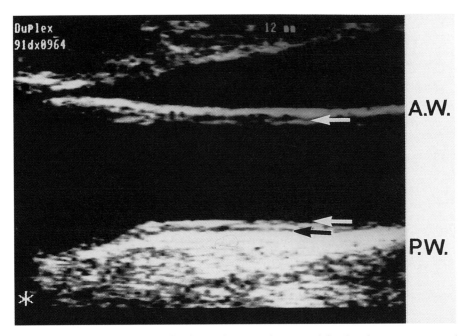

Figure 2. Characteristic longitudinal 2-D ultrasound image of the distal common carotid artery. AW = Anterior (near) wall of the carotid artery ; PW = Posterior (far) wall of the carotid artery. Arrows from top to bottom indicate the leading edge of the intima-lumen interface at the near wall, the lumen-intima interfaces and the media-adventitia interface at the far wall, respectively.

According to the 'leading edge principle' the distance of the leading edge of the first bright line of the far wall (lumen-intima interface) and the leading edge of the second bright line (media-adventitia interface) indicates the intima-media thickness of the far wall of the distal common carotid artery (24). With respect to the near wall the distance of the trailing edge of the first bright line of the near wall and the trailing edge of the second bright line is probably the best estimate of the intima-media thickness of the near wall (19).

In most studies the entire session or part of the ultrasound examination of the carotid arteries is recorded on videotape, and intima-media thickness is measured off-line from the recorded images using specialized dedicated computer software.

B. Near Wall and Far Wall

Validation studies have compared the precise location of the interfaces as seen with high resolution B-mode ultrasound with the histologic layers of the arterial wall (19,24,25). This topic is discussed elsewhere.

The near wall findings in the validation studies have lead to an intensive discussion on whether near wall intima-media measurements should be performed at all. Results from the Rotterdam Study have indicated that the association between near wall intima-media thickness and prevalent cardiovascular disease is as strong and precise as compared to the association found for the far wall. Combining information of the near wall and far wall common carotid intima-media thickness into one intima-media thickness estimate (average of four sites) provided the strongest association with cardiovascular disease in this study (Bots ML, Unpublished data). In addition, findings in three randomized placebo controlled intervention studies among subjects receiving placebo treatment indicated that the progression rate of near wall common carotid intima-media thickness was similar to that for the far wall common carotid intima-media thickness (26). Furthermore, combining information of both near and far wall yielded estimates of progression rates with higher precision, i.e., smaller standard errors. Clearly, measurement of near wall intima-media thickness yields valuable information, and should not be discarded easily in population-based studies on atherosclerosis (26). Of course, standardization of gain settings and B-mode ultrasound technique across various sonographers is of utmost importance.

C. Quantifying Carotid Atherosclerosis Using Intima-Media Thickness

Currently, several non-invasive ultrasound protocols are being used to quantify the presence and extent of carotid atherosclerosis. In general, these approaches differ in four aspects, i.e., the length of the segment of the measurement (maximum or mean intima-media thickness); the artery (left or right); the site (common carotid artery, carotid bifurcation and internal carotid artery) and the location of the measurement (near and far wall). Similarly, the individual outcome variable, based on intima-media thickness measurements, differs across studies from an average of all measurements at all sites and locations to site specific far wall measurements. Few have used centiles of the distribution of the site specific intima-media thickness measurements to characterize subjects with and without carotid atherosclerosis.

The correlation between maximum intima-media thickness and mean intima-media thickness is very high ($r=0.88$) (26). Studies in which information of both parameters is available have shown similar associations with respect to direction and strength for maximum and mean intima-media thickness with cardiovascular risk factors and prevalent cardiovascular disease. It has been suggested to use the average intima-media thickness, measured at predefined segments as an indicator of extent of carotid atherosclerosis, and use the maximum intima-media thickness as an estimate of severity of carotid atherosclerosis (27).

There is no reason to believe that the association between intima-media thickness and cardiovascular disease or atherosclerosis elsewhere in the arterial system would differ between the right and the left carotid artery. Indeed, several studies have shown similar results with respect to magnitude and precision of these associations (26). Results from the Cardiovascular Health Study indicated slightly stronger associations for internal carotid intima-media thickness with prevalent coronary heart disease compared to common carotid intima-media thickness (28). For stroke associations were stronger for common carotid intima-media thickness compared to internal carotid intima-media thickness. It should be recognized that, in general, internal carotid intima-media thickness measurements are more difficult to obtain than common carotid intima-media thickness measurements. Combining the information obtained from both near and far wall of the common carotid artery, the carotid bifurcation and the internal carotid artery at both left and right side results in an estimate for carotid atherosclerosis with enhanced precision. Consequently, due to the increased precision of the measurement, the magnitude of the association under study would increase (26).

Differences in quantifying presence and extent of carotid atherosclerosis across studies should be appreciated. At present, however, it can not be answered satisfactory which approach provides the 'best' indicator of atherosclerosis for cross-sectional studies, for assessment of change over time, and for studies on determinants of progression of intima-media thickness.

IV. MAIN FINDINGS OF POPULATION-BASED STUDIES

A. Cross-sectional Results

Several studies demonstrated that with increasing age common carotid intima-media thickness increases in both men and women. The estimates of change in common carotid intima-media thickness based on cross-sectional data were around 0.009 mm/yr for men and women (28-30). Common carotid intima-media thickness was increased in men compared to women for all ages, with a mean difference of around 5 to 10 %. Although this may reflect a difference in atherosclerotic status, it may also be that normal artery intima-media thickness is greater in men than in women. Elevated levels of established cardiovascular risk factors, such as LDL cholesterol, systolic blood pressure, body mass index, and a decrease in HDL cholesterol were associated with an increased intima-media thickness (14,16,18,28). As an example, results from the ARIC study are presented in table 2. Additionally, subjects with presence of hypertension, smoking and diabetes mellitus have an increased carotid intima-media thickness compared to subjects without these conditions (14,16,18,28,31-3). Results from the Cardiovascular Health Study and the Rotterdam Study indicated an increase in intima-media thickness of about 8 % among subjects with hypertension compared to normotensive subjects (28). For current smoking the increase in intima-media thickness was between 5 and 10 % increased relative to non-smokers (34). The magnitude of the difference in intima-media thickness in subjects with diabetes mellitus compared to subjects without glucose intolerance ranged from 7 to 12 %.

Increase intake of dietary components of supposed atherogenic and antiatherogenic properties has been related to carotid intima-media thickness. Results from the ARIC study have shown that increased intake of animal fat, saturated fat, mono-unsaturated fat, and cholesterol were positively associated with carotid wall thickness, whereas an inverse relation was found for vegetable fat intake and polyunsaturated fat intake (35). Similarly, increased intake of antioxidants (β-carotene and vitamin A) was found to be related to a reduced carotid intima-media thickness (36). This observation is consistent with earlier findings of Salonen and co-workers indicating that factors involved in oxidative modification of LDL cholesterol, such as serum copper and selenium, were associated with a reduced progression of intima-media thickness (37).

Table 2. Associations between carotid atherosclerosis and cardiovascular risk factors. Findings from the ARIC study.

Risk factor	mean cases	mean controls	mean diff.	S.E. diff.
Age (years)	56.8	55.5	1.27	0.20
Body mass index (kg/m²)	26.9	26.3	0.65	0.31
Systolic blood pressure (mmHg)	127.9	117.5	10.41	1.27
Diastolic blood pressure (mmHg)	74.2	72.2	1.99	0.75
Cigarette smoking (pack-years)	29.1	14.1	14.99	1.71
Total cholesterol (mg/dl)	225.6	207.8	17.71	2.91
LDL cholesterol (mg/dl)	146.7	129.8	16.90	2.90
HDL cholesterol (mg/dl)	49.9	55.4	-5.53	1.18
Total triglyceride (mg/dl)	144.7	113.7	31.01	5.58

HDL = high density lipoprotein; LDL = low density lipoprotein.
All p < 0.05

At present limited information is present on the association between coagulation factors, such as fibrinogen, factor VII activity and factor VIII activity, and intima-media thickness. Elevated levels of fibrinogen were related to increased intima-media independent of other established cardiovascular risk factors (16,38-9). Factor VII activity was positively associated with increased intima-media thickness in univariate analyses in the ARIC study, but after adjustment for differences in cardiovascular risk factors, the association lost its significance (38). Indicators of platelet activity, such as beta-thromboglobulin level, and markers for reduced fibrinolysis, such as increased PAI-1 levels, have been associated with increased intima-media thickness (40-1). Results from other studies, however, are awaited.

Subjects with prevalent cardiovascular disease, such as myocardial infarction, angina pectoris, intermittent claudication and stroke, have in general a thicker common carotid intima-media compared to those without symptomatic cardiovascular disease. The magnitude of the difference in common carotid intima-media thickness between subjects with and without symptomatic cardiovascular disease varies from 6 to 12 % across studies (42-4). Findings from the Cardiovascular Health Study showed slightly stronger studies (42-4). Findings from the Cardiovascular Health Study showed slightly stronger associations between common carotid intima-media thickness and prevalent stroke compared to internal carotid intima-media thickness (28). For coronary heart disease the reverse was true (Figure 3). In addition, common carotid intima-media thickness has been reported to be strongly related to left ventricular mass, measured by echocardiography (31,45-7).

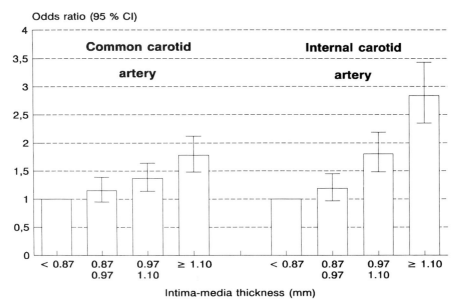

Figure 3. Association between carotid intima-media thickness and coronary heart disease. Results from the Cardiovascular Health Study (28).

An increased common carotid intima-media thickness has been shown to be associated with presence of atherosclerosis elsewhere in the arterial system. Subjects with atherosclerotic abnormalities in the carotid bifurcation or internal carotid artery had an increased common carotid intima-media thickness compared with those without abnormalities (29,42,48). Furthermore, presence of calcifications of the abdominal aorta was associated with an 18 % increase in common carotid intima-media thickness (49).

Results from the Rotterdam Study have demonstrated a gradual association between the increase in common carotid intima-media thickness and a decrease in ankle-arm index, i.e., an indicator of atherosclerosis in the arteries of the lower extremities (Figure 4) (20).

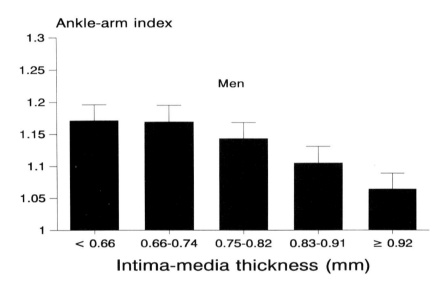

Adjusted for age

Figure 4. Association between intima-media thickness and ankle-arm index. Results from the Rotterdam study (20)

B. Longitudinal Results

Longitudinal results can be roughly categorized into three groups: intima-media thickness as a predictor of future cardiovascular disease; change of intima-media thickness over time; intima-media thickness as a major outcome measure(atherosclerosis endpoint) in studies in which baseline risk factors were collected long before ultrasonography of the carotid arteries was performed.

At present, results on intima-media thickness as a predictor of cardiovascular disease are sparse. This is mainly due to the limited follow-up time of the existing observational studies. Salonen and co-workers in the Kuopio Ischemic Heart Disease Risk Factor study found that an increase in intima-media thickness of 0.1 mm was associated with an increased risk of myocardial infarction of 11 % [95 % C.I. 6,16] (50). Preliminary findings from the ARIC study, presented at the Third Conference on Preventive Cardiology in Oslo, Norway in 1993, indicated a strong association between intima-media thickness and incident myocardial infarction. The first results from the Rotterdam Study using 26 medically confirmed myocardial infarctions, indicated that with an increase of 0.1 mm in common carotid intima-media thickness the risk of a myocardial infarction increased 35 % (R.R. 1.35; 95 % C.I.: 1.10, 1.60).

Although the limited information on this issue is consistent across studies, in the near future these findings will be augmented with results from analyses with a larger number of events, providing more stable estimates of future risk associated with the level of carotid intima-media thickness at baseline.

Data   on change over time in intima-media thickness and its determinants are limited. Salonen and co-workers reported that smoking and increased LDL cholesterol are strongly associated with increase in intima-media thickness over time in Eastern Finnish men (51). Information on the association between progression of carotid intima-media thickness and risk of cardiovascular disease is presently virtually absent. Most of the current information on change in intima-media thickness over time comes from analyses on data of subjects in placebo groups in intervention studies (51-5). The estimates of progression rates differs considerably across studies. The observed changes over time per year in intima-media thickness were 0.027 mm in ACAPS, 0.05mm in CLASS, and 0.09mm, in KAPS, and 0.027 mm in PLACII. Further information will be discussed in the chapter discussing the Clinical Trials. Differences in the used methodology, in outcome measure, and in selection of participants may at least partly explain the differences in estimates of progression rates of carotid intima-media thickness. In studies on estimating progression in intima-media thickness over time several aspects need to be considered that may be great importance to the observed findings. This includes random and systematic differences across subjects who measure intima-media thickness from the stored images on videotape (readers). Considerable differences may be present as has been exemplified by Furberg and co-workers (26). Furthermore, reader behavior within the same person may change over time from initially reading 'thick' to ultimately reading 'thin' or vice versa. The magnitude of these differences, despite strict quality control efforts may be as large as 0.1 mm (26). To some extent mortality during follow-up may bias progression rates towards a lower estimate, assuming an increased risk of death among those who progress rapidly.

Finally, some observational studies have been performed using carotid intima-media thickness measurements as the major outcome. In these studies the association between cardiovascular risk factors, collected long before ultrasonography of the carotid arteries was performed, and intima-media thickness was studied. In elderly Finnish men smoking, increased LDL cholesterol level, and an increased pulse pressure measured in 1959 were significantly associated with carotid atherosclerosis measured in 1989 (44). Joensuu and co-workers in a study in which nine months after risk factor measurements, ultrasonography of carotid and femoral arteries was performed, showed that systolic blood pressure, total cholesterol, age and pack-years of smoking were the most important determinants of common carotid intima-media thickness (56).

V. CONCLUSION

Intima-media thickness measurement provides an exiting potential for non-invasive research on atherosclerosis. The relation between carotid intima-media thickness and various cardiovascular risk factors is well established in cross-sectional studies. Future results from currently ongoing observational studies will provide information on the value of carotid intima-media thickness as predictor of incident cardiovascular disease, such as myocardial infraction, angina pectoris and stroke. Furthermore, studies on estimates and determinants of progression of carotid intima-media thickness and the relation between increased progression rates and the risk of cardiovascular disease are well under way. It is the length of the follow-up time which, at this moment, has been the most limiting factor for results to emerge. These results may lead to identification of factors that are potentially suitable to intervene upon in order to prevent symptomatic cardiovascular disease (29).

Finally, non-invasive assessment of atherosclerosis opens new areas of research, and enables us to study more directly in the population at large the association between atherosclerosis and other disease processes, such as for example the association between atherosclerosis and decline in cognitive function or between atherosclerosis and ophthalmologic diseases such as age related macula degeneration (57-9).

References

1.   Thom TJ. International mortality from heart disease: Rates and trends. Int J Epidemiol 1989; 18 (suppl 1): S20-8.
2.   Oliver MF. Prevention of coronary heart disease: Propaganda, promises, problems and prospects. Circulation 1986;73:1-9.
3   Muller JE, Tofler GH, Stone PH. Circadian variation and triggers of onset of acute cardiovascular disease. Circulation 1989;79:733-43.
4.   Willich SN, Goldberg RJ, Maclure M, Perriello L, Muller JE. Increased onset of sudden cardiac death in the first three hours after awakening. Am J Cardiol 1992;70:65-8.
5.   Andreotti F, Davies GJ, Hackett DR, et al. Major circadian fluctuations in fibrinolytic factors and possible relevance to time of onset of myocardial infarction, sudden death and stroke. Am J Cardiol 1988;62:635-7.
6.   Ridker PM, Manson JE, Goldhaber SZ, Hennekens CH, Buring JE. Comparison of delay times of hospital presentation for physicians and nonphysicians with acute myocardial infarction. Am J Cardiol 1992;70: 10-3.
7.   Vogt MT, Wolfson SK, Kuller LH. Lower extremity arterial disease and the ageing process: A review. J Clin Epidemiol 1992;45:529-42.
8.   Witteman JCM, Grobbee DE, Kok FJ, Hofman A, Valkenburg HA. Increased risk of atherosclerosis in women after the menopause Br Med J 1989;298:642-5.
9.   Witteman JCM, Kok FJ, Saase JLCM van, Valkenburg HA. Aortic calcification as a predictor of cardiovascular mortality. Lancet 1986;ii: 1120-2.
10. Witteman JCM, Grobbee DE, Valkenburg HA, et al. A J-shaped relation between change in diastolic blood pressure and progression of aortic atherosclerosis. Lancet 1994;343:504-07.
11. Wong ND, Vo A, Abrahamson D, Tobis JM, Eisenberg H, Detrano RC. Detection of coronary artery calcium by ultrafast computed tomography and its relation to clinical evidence of coronary artery disease. Am J Cardiol 1994;73:223-7
12. Wong ND, Kouwabunpat D, Vo AN, et al. Coronary calcium and atherosclerosis by ultrafast computed tomography in asymptomatic men and women: relation to age and risk factors. Am Heart J 1994; 127:422-30.
13. Merickel MB, Berr S, Spetz K, et al. Noninvasive quantitative evaluation of atherosclerosis using MRI and image analysis. Arterioscler Thromb 1993; 1180-6.
14. Heiss G, Sharett AR, Barnes R, Chambles LE, Szklo M, Alzola C. Carotid atherosclerosis measured by B-mode ultrasound in populations: Associations with cardiovascular risk factors in the ARIC study. Am J Epidemiol 1991; 134:250-6.
15. O'Leary DH, Polak JF, Wolfson SK, et al. Use of sonography to evaluate carotid atherosclerosis in the elderly. The Cardiovascular Health Study. Stroke 1991;22:1155-63.
16. Salonen R, Salonen JT. Determinants of carotid intima-media thickness: A population-based ultrasonography study in eastern Finnish men. J Int Med 1991;229:225-31.
17. Wendethag 1, Olov G, Wikstrand J. Arterial wall thickness in familial hypercholesterolemia. Ultrasound measurements of intima-media thickness in the common carotid artery. Arterioscler Thromb 1992; 12:70-7.
18. Bots ML, Hofman A, Bruyn AM de, Jong PTVM de, Grobbee De. Isolated systolic hypertension and vessel wall thickness of the carotid artery: The Rotterdam Study. Arterioscler Thromb 1993; 13:64-9.
19. Wendelhag I, Gustavsson T, Suurkiila M, Berglund G, Wikstrand J. Ultrasound measurement of wall thickness in the carotid artery: Fundamental principles, and description of a computerized analyzing system. Clin Physiol 1991; 1 1:565-77.
20. Bots ML, Hofman A, Grobbee DE. Common carotid intima-media thickness and lower extremity arterial atherosclerosis. The Rotterdam Study. Arterioscler Thromb 1994;14:1885-91
21. Willeit J, Kiechl S. Prevalence and risk factors of asymptomatic extracranial carotid artery atherosclerosis. A population-based study. Arterioscler Thromb 1993; 13:661-8.
22. Prati P, Vanuzzo D, Casaroli M, et al. Prevalence and determinants of carotid atherosclerosis in a general population. Stroke 1992;23:1705-11.
23. Bonithon-Kopp C, Scarabin P, Taquet A, Touboul P, Malmejac A, Guize L. Risk factors for early carotid atherosclerosis in middle-aged French women. Arteriosclerosis and Thrombosis 1991; 11: 966-972.
24. Pignoli P, Tremoli E, Poli A, Oreste P, Paoletti R. Intimal plus medial thickness of the arterial wall: A direct measurement with ultrasound imaging. Circulation 1986;74:1399-1406.
25. Wong M, Edelstein J, Wollman J, Bond MG. Ultrasonic-pathological comparison of the human arterial wall. Verification of intima-media thickness. Arteriosl Thromb 1993; 13:482-6.
26. Furberg CD, Byington RP, Craven TE. Lessons learned from clinical trials with ultrasound endpoints. J Int Med 1994;236:575-80.
27. Espeland MA, Hoen H, Byington R, Howard G, Riley WA, Furberg CD. Spatial distribution of carotid intimal-medial thickness as measured by B-mode ultrasonography. Stroke 1994;25:1812-19.

28. O'Leary DH, Polak JF, Kronmal RA, et al. Distribution and correlates of sonographically detected carotid artery disease in the Cardiovascular Health Study. Stroke 1992;23:1752-60.
29. Grobbee DE, Bots ML. Carotid artery intima-media thickness as an indicator of generalized atherosclerosis. J Int Med 1994;236:567-73.
30. Howard G, Sharrett AR, Heiss G, et al. Carotid artery intimal-medial thickness distribution in general populations as evaluated by B-mode ultrasound. Stroke 1993;24:1297-1304.
31. Psaty BM, Furberg CD, Kuller LH, et al. Isolated systolic hypertension and subclinical cardiovascular disease in the elderly. Initial findings from the Cardiovascular Health Study. JAMA 1992;268:1287-9.
32. Folsom AR, Eckfeldt JH, Weitzman, et al. Relation of carotid artery wall thickness to diabetes mellitus, fasting glucose and insulin, body size, and physical activity. Stroke 1994;25:66-73.
33. Salonen R, Salonen JT. Carotid atherosclerosis in relation to systolic and diastolic blood pressure: Kuopio ischaemic heart disease risk factor study. Ann Med 1991;23:23-7.
34. Salonen JT, Salonen R. Ultrasound B-mode imaging in observational studies of atherosclerotic progression. Circulation 1993;87 (suppl II):56-65.
35. Tell GS, Evans GW, Folsom AR, Shimakaw T, Carpenter MA, Heiss G. Dietary fat intake and carotid artery wall thickness. The Atherosclerosis Risk in Communities (ARIC) study. Am J Epidemiol 1994;139:979-89.
36. Kritechevsky SB, Shimakawa T, Dennis B, et al. Dietary antioxidants and carotid intima-media wall thickness: The ARIC study (abstract). Circulation 1993;87:679.
37. Salonen JT, Salonen R, Seppinen K, et al. Interactions of serum copper, selenium and low density lipoprotein cholesterol in atherogenesis. Br Med J 1991;302:756-60.
38. Folsom AR, Wu KK, Shahar E, Davis CE. Association of hemostatic variables with prevalent cardiovascular disease and asymptomatic carotid artery atherosclerosis. Arterioscler Thromb 1993; 13:1829-36.
39. Bots ML, Breslau PJ, Briet E, de Bruin AM, van Vliet HH, van der Ouweland FA, de Jong PT, Hofman A, Grobbee DE. Cardiovascular determinants of carotid artery disease. The Rotterdam Elderly Study. Hypertension 1992;19:717-20
40. Cortes J, Salomaa VV, Heiss G, et al. In-vivo platelet activation and asymptomatic atherosclerosis. The Atherosclerosis Risk In Communities (ARIC) study, 19861989. (abstract). Circulation 1993;87:698.
41. Salomaa VV, Wu KK, Stinson VL, et al. The association of fibrinolytic activity with asymptomatic carotid atherosclerosis: The ARIC study. (abstract) Circulation 1993;87:699.
42. Polak JF, O'Leary DH, Kronmal RA, et al. Sonographic evaluation of the carotid artery atherosclerosis in the elderly: Relationship of disease severity to stroke and transient ischemic attack. Radiology 1993; 188:363-70.
43. Bots ML, Hofman A, Grobbee DE. Common carotid intima-media thickness and cardiovascular disease in the Rotterdam Study. A cross-sectional analysis. In: W Koenig, V Hombach, MG Bond, and DM Kramsh, Eds. Progression and Regression of Atherosclerosis. Blackwell Wissenschaft, Wien, 1995, pp.118-23
44. Salonen R, Tervahauta M, Salonen JT, Pekkanen J, Nissinen A, Karvonen MJ. Ultrasonographic manifestations of common carotid atherosclerosis in elderly Eastern Finnish men. Arterioscler Thromb 1994; 14:1631-40.
45. Roman MJ, Saba PS, Pini R, et al. Parallel cardiac and vascular adaptation in hypertension. Circulation 1992;86:1909-18.
46. Hughes AD, Sinclair AM, Geroulakos G, et al. Structural changes in the hearts and carotid arteries associated with hypertension in humans. J Hum Hypertension 1993;7:395-7.
47. Bots ML, Mosterd A, Hong Y, Grobbee DE. Increased common carotid intima media thickness and increased left ventricular mass in a population-based study. The Rotterdam Study. (Abstract). Joint XIIth world congress of cardiology and XVIth European Society of Cardiology. Berlin, Germany 1994.
48. Howard G, Burke GL, Evans GW, et al. Relations of intimal-medial thickness among sites within the carotid artery as evaluated by B-mode ultrasound. The Atherosclerosis Risk in Communities study. Stroke 1994;25:1581-7.
49. Bots ML, Witteman JCM, Grobbee DE. Carotid intima-media wall thickness in elderly women with and without atherosclerosis of the abdominal aorta. Atherosclerosis 1993; 102:99-105.
50. Salonen JT, Salonen R. Ultrasonographically assessed carotid morphology and the risk of coronary heart disease. Arterioscler Thromb 1991; 11:1245-9.
51. Salonen R, Salonen JT. Progression of carotid atherosclerosis and its determinants: A population-based ultrasonography study. Atherosclerosis 1990;81:33-40.
52. Blankenhorn DH, Selzer RH, Crawford DW, et al. Beneficial effects of colestipol-niacin therapy on the common carotid artery. Circulation 1993;88:20-8.
53. Furberg CD, Adams HP, Applegate WB, et al. Effect of lovastatin on early carotid atherosclerosis and cardiovascular events. Circulation 1994;90:1679-87.

54. Crouse JR, Byington RP, Bond MG, et al. Pravastatin, lipids and atherosclerosis in the carotid arteries: design features of a clinical trial with carotid atherosclerosis outcome. Control Clin Trials 1992; 13:495-506.

55. Salonen JT, Salonen R. Risk factors for carotid and femoral atherosclerosis in hypercholesterolaemic men. J Int Med 1994;236:561-6.

56. Joensuu T, Salonen R, Winblad I, Korpela H, Salonen JT. Determinants of femoral and carotid artery atherosclerosis. J Int Med 1994;236:799-84.

57. Bots ML, VanSwieten J, Breteler MMB, DeJong PTVM, Pols HP, VanGijn J, Hofman A, Grobbee DE. Cerebral white matter lesions and atherosclerosis in the Rotterdam Study. Lancet 1993;341:1232-7.

58. Breteler MMB, Claus JJ, Grobbee DE, Hofman A. Cardiovascular disease and distribution of cognitive function in elderly people. The Rotterdam Study. Br Med J 1994;308:1604-8.

59. Vingerling JR, Dielemans I, Bots ML, Hofman A, Grobbee DE, Jong PTVM de. Age-related macular degeneration is associated with atherosclerosis. The Rotterdam Study. Am J Epidemiol 1995;142:404-9.

INTERVENTIONAL CLINICAL TRIALS ON CAROTID ATHEROSCLEROSIS PROGRESSION

Michele Mercuri, M.D., Ph.D. Rong Tang, M.D. and M. Gene Bond, Ph.D.

Bowman Gray School of Medicine of Wake Forest University
Winston-Salem, North Carolina U.S.A.

Contents

I. RATIONALE FOR INTERVENTIONAL CLINICAL TRIALS

The intrinsic links between morphologic manifestations of atherosclerosis and their clinical sequelae stress the importance of preventing the action of major cardiovascular risk factors in the initiation, progression and complication of atherosclerotic plaques. By focusing on prevention, the natural targets of the investigations are no longer and exclusively the survivors of acute ischemic events and/or symptomatic patients with advanced disease, but also, and most importantly the asymptomatic young-adults with a genetic predisposition or a high risk factor profile for cardiovascular disease. Targeting this segment of population requires innovative, non-invasive diagnostic techniques ranging from sophisticated epidemiological surveys to quantitative imaging methodologies.

Metanalytical interpretations and the main results of the two most recent and largest clinical trials testing the effects of HMGCoA reductase inhibitors on total and cardiovascular morbidity and mortality of asymptomatic (1) and symptomatic (2,3) patients with moderate to high LDL-cholesterol levels have provided direct evidences that prevention of coronary events is feasible and achievable through specific pharmacological intervention. These trials showed that the efficacy of these hypocholesterolemic drugs is significant, and when patients at high risk are treated continuously for up to five years there is a 0.3 or more reduction in cardiovascular events, and a similar reduction in total mortality. However, data from the WOSCOPS (1), a primary prevention clinical trial, showed that after five years, the absolute risk for coronary events in 35 to 65 year old patients with hypercholesterolemia, is 0.1, and that treatment with pravastatin reduces this risk to 0.07. These results suggest that clinical trials target a population affected by a wide range of atherosclerosis extent and severity, and the asymptomatic status, as currently defined for clinical purposes, is probably an inefficient criterion to characterize primary prevention for at least two reasons. First because economic necessity will unlikely allow to extend expensive treatments to a large segment of the population affected by moderate hypercholesterolemia. Second because, despite the treatment, over 0.7 of the population at true risk for the occurrence of an event within 5 years does not benefit from the treatment. The most compelling question rising from these data regards the criteria to be used in selecting the patients who will benefit from these treatments. If in fact the potential treatment benefit, as shown by the significant reduction in the 5 year risk, attains to 0.1 of the population selected on the basis of their LDL-cholesterol levels, which are the specific criteria we should use to better characterize the population at risk? Sufficient data are not available to operationally react to this question. Therefore , it is necessary to investigate the mechanisms through which pharmacological intervention provides cardiovascular protection, to define screening methodologies, to supplement laboratory techniques and traditional risk factor analysis, which will be able to better characterize patients' risk.

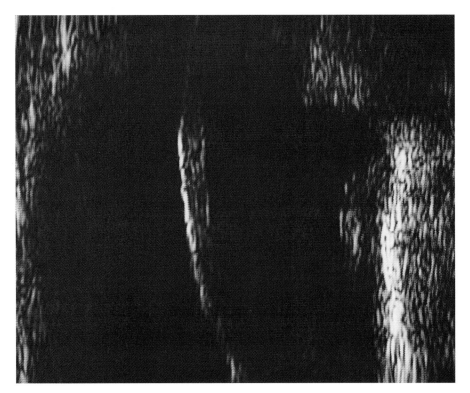

Figure 1. B-mode ultrasound imaging of the bifurcation carotid artery. An atherosclerotic plaque is imaged on the far wall (1.45mm). [Biosound 2000 II s.a., 8 M Hz].

Quantitative B-mode ultrasound imaging protocols provide an excellent methodology to be used in interventional clinical trials. B-mode ultrasound can supplement and support traditional procedures used for risk stratification. B-mode ultrasound is totally risk free, relatively inexpensive and provide direct information on the morphological characteristics of peripheral arteries which (Figure 1) have been correlated to prevalence of atherosclerosis, major cardiovascular risk factors and coronary artery disease status. This non invasive technique offers an excellent opportunity to test, in asymptomatic subjects at risk for cardiovascular diseases, the effects of different pharmacological treatments. In particular it would be possible to determine whether drug benefits come from a direct effect on specific components of the arterial wall (arterial thickness and/or stenosis) and/or atherosclerotic plaques (structure) and/or vascular reactivity and remodeling (function).

In the last 15 years, ultrasound researchers have been focusing their attention to the standardization of quantitative protocols aimed at detecting and monitoring carotid arterial walls as expressed by changes in intima media thicknesses (IMT). This surrogate endpoint is being used worldwide, and it is the current standard for interventional clinical trials in primary prevention settings to test the effects of HMGCoA reductase inhibitors, calcium antagonists, α-, β-, and ACE-Inhibitors (4).

II.   ENDPOINTS FOR CONTROLLED CLINICAL TRIALS OF ATHEROSCLEROSIS

The specific definition of the endpoints used in a controlled clinical trial of atherosclerosis is of critical importance especially for the interpretation of the study results and across study comparison.

A consistent amount of data acquired in different laboratories show that B-mode ultrasound imaging is a valid surrogate measurement of atherosclerosis histologically and epidemiologically (see previous chapters). However, a methodological standardization across laboratory is still lacking.

It is largely agreed upon that the IMT must be measured as the linear distance, perpendicular to the arterial wall, which goes from the ultrasonic boundary between lumen and intima to the boundary between media and adventitia. The principle inter-laboratory differences fall on 4 main issues: near vs. far wall measurements, whether the IMT should be measured at the plaque site, the handling of missing data, and the number of arterial segments to be included in the calculation of the surrogate endpoints.

Some of the issues above were discussed in the previous chapters, but it is relevant to reaffirm here that since this technique is relatively new, and more data are still required before recommendations can be largely agreed upon, whenever reporting the results of studies using B-mode ultrasound, the methods used should be carefully described in great detail to allow across study comparisons (5).

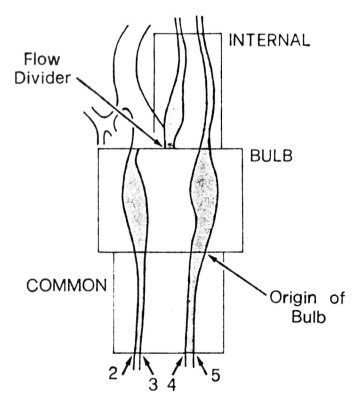

Figure 2. Schematic diagram showing the three segments of the right carotid artery, the two anatomic landmarks used to standardize wall registration (flow divider and origin of the bulb), and the specific B-mode ultrasound interfaces used to calculate the intima media thicknesses (2 and 5 are the media adventitia boundaries, 3 and 4 the lumen intima boundaries, 2 to 3 the near wall intima media thickness, and 4 to 5 the far wall intima media thickness).

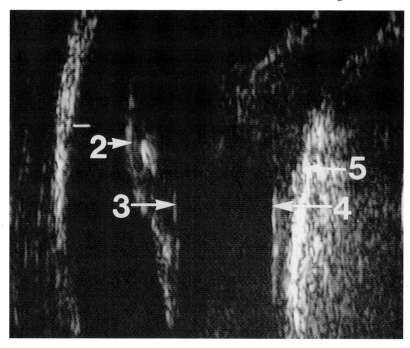

Figure 3. B-mode ultrasound imaging of the carotid artery bifurcation showing intima media thickening on both near and far walls. [Biosound 2000 II s.a., 8 M Hz]

In the majority of clinical trials reported so far, the three endpoints chosen are often the Mean Maximum IMT (MMax), the Far Wall Common and Bifurcation IMT (CBFMax) and Single Maximum IMT (TMax or 1st Max). The basic ultrasonographic elements which define the above outcome measurements are shown in Figure 2 and 3. The MMax is defined as the mean of the individual maximum IMT detected in up to 12 standardized carotid segments (Carotid Mean Maximum IMT or MMax) including the near and far walls of the distal cm of the common carotid artery, the carotid bulb and the proximal cm of the internal carotid artery bilaterally. The CBFMax is a variation of the MMax in which only the maximum IMT of four walls, i.e., the far wall of the common and bifurcation bilaterally, are taken into consideration. MMax and CBFMax were designed to estimate the extent and severity of carotid atherosclerosis. The TMax is the single maximum IMT detected across the entire arterial section examined during the ultrasound study and was chosen to estimate the thickest atherosclerotic plaque.

In general, the analysis plan (6-9) includes the estimate of the individual patient aggregate IMT slope of progression, which is computed by taking into consideration each individual   patient's visit aggregate measurements and calculated by fitting these points into a regression model weighed for the time and number of visits, the baseline aggregate IMT and other significant   covariables. The individual regressions are then used to calculate the mean treatment group slopes, i.e., the "b" of the regression equation. Then, group comparisons are made using appropriate statistics. Several factors affect the power of such perspective studies aimed at detecting treatment efficacy and involving serial measurements of surrogate endpoints. From a theoretical point of view, the variance in estimating the group slope, i.e., *variance (b)*, is given by the interpatient variability, is directly related to the square of the measurement error and inversely related to the number and timing of visits. Therefore, the balance between and among these variables is the key to insure proper testing of regression hypothesis. In general, and without entering sophisticated mathematics, it seems that an interventional clinical trial using ultrasound outcome measurements requires a follow up of no less than 3 years and a minimum of 6 visits equally distributed across the study period. Furthermore, the measurement error should be kept under an absolute difference in replicate scans of 0.1mm or less. Under these assumptions, a trial with two treatment groups may be performed with a minimum of 300 patients (10).

It is also important to underline that the *intention to treat approach*, and a procedure for adjusting the statistical significance to multiple comparisons must be part of the standard *per* protocol analysis. In fact, in prospective investigation involving new treatments for chronic diseases, patients' withdrawal and side effects condition the drop out rates and affect the availability of complete data sets. These drop outs and data missingness may represent intolerance to treatment, and/or the presence of unrecognized side effects. Furthermore, since the use of multiple endpoints is common in these trials, after choosing the primary and secondary outcome measurements, it is important to avoid the occurrence of chance results. These two analytical features must be part of any standard protocol.

III.   CLINICAL TRIALS WITH ANTIHYPERTENSIVE DRUGS.

Hypertension is directly and indirectly related to morphological changes of endothelial and smooth muscle cells, interacts with other cardiovascular risk factors, and is a major contributor to the development of atherosclerotic plaques (11). Furthermore, it has been shown that blood pressure control reduces cerebrovascular ischemic deaths and improves CHD survival (12). However, traditional drug treatment, i.e. , diuretic and ß-blockers, failed to provide a similar protection against CHD mortality as seen in cerebrovascular accidents (13). In a strive to improve the efficacy of antihypertensive drugson target organ disease, researchers have discovered that calcium antagonists and ACE inhibitors affect several key atherogenic elements, i.e., smooth muscle cells, endothelial function, growth factors, and matrix production (14). In addition, these compounds show the ability to reduce the incidence of atherosclerosis in animal models (15). A few secondary prevention clinical trials were performed in patients with established CHD, and using quantitative coronary arteriographic endpoints (16,17). The results of the INTACT and MHIS suggested that calcium antagonists may have an effect on early lesions and on new lesion development. However, the results of these trials were inconclusive, and led to the search for new ways to prove the efficacy of calcium antagonists and ACE inhibitors on atherosclerosis. B-mode ultrasound imaging endpoints seemed to offer the opportunity for testing additional hypotheses especially in the area of early disease.

IV. THE MULTICENTER ISRADIPINE/DIURETIC ATHEROSCLEROSIS STUDY

Without doubts, most of the credit for the recent popularity of interventional clinical trials using ultrasound based surrogate endpoints must be given to the researchers who designed the Multicenter Isradipine/Diuretic Atherosclerosis Study (MIDAS) (18-19). MIDAS presented a very innovative approach to test the morphologic effects of pharmacological treatment of atherosclerosis. All clinical trialists, who subsequently became involved with this kind of research learned and are benefiting from the experiences presented and debated by the MIDAS research group (20).

MIDAS was the first interventional primary prevention clinical trial in hypertension using surrogate endpoints clearly related to plaque progression. Contrary to the clinical trials testing the efficacy of lipid lowering drugs, trials on patients with hypertension require an active treatment control. Therefore, in these trial category the research hypothesis is to determine whether one specific drug offers any advantage over a standard and/or less expensive treatment provided that both are equally effective in controlling the patients' blood pressure.

In MIDAS, the objective was to assess the efficacy of isradipine, a calcium antagonist, and hydrochlorothiazide (HCTZ), a diuretic, in reducing the progression of early carotid atherosclerosis. In addition, the trial aimed at determining the treatment effects on lipid profiles, left ventricular mass, clinical cardiovascular events, and quality of life. Eight hundred 83 hypertensive patients (mean age 58.5 years, 0.78 men, 0.39 smokers, LDL-cholesterol: 146mg/dL) with a diastolic blood pressure in the range of 90-115 mmHg (mean 96.5 mmHg), and asymptomatic carotid lesions (1.3<TMax<3.5 mm) participated in the 3 year prospective study. They received isradipine 2.5-5 mg, or HCTZ 12.5-25 mg, twice daily; if this regimen did not normalize their diastolic blood pressure, enalapril, an ACE inhibitor, was given open label. The primary endpoint for the study was the MMax (baseline MMax 1.17 mm), the outcome measure was the difference in the three year slope of progression in the two treatment groups. Standardized ultrasound examinations were performed at baseline, just before starting the treatment, and then semiannually for up to three years. Image processing stations were used by certified readers to quantitate each patient's visit carotid ultrasound measurements. MIDAS was the first trial to design and implement a protocol for a standardized quality control assessment. The key feature of this protocol was to replicate baseline and 36 month follow up scans and reading. This set of data were then used to calculate cross sectional variations in measurements reproducibility (19), and to increase the precision in estimating the patients' MMax progression.

Briefly, MIDAS final ultrasound findings show (8) that the progression of carotid MMax is slower in hypertensives treated with isradipine when compared to HCTZ. However, this difference is not significant and does not result from an interaction between treatment and time. In fact, the difference between isradipine and HCTZ was observed early in the follow up, and continued to the end of the study without further increases, i.e., the two group regression curves did not further diverge as a result of the treatment. This finding does not prove any significant advantage of isradipine over HCTZ in controlling the progression of carotid IMT.

The interpretation of the results were complicated by the observation that the progression did not fit a linear model, therefore an alternative statistical model to the original *per* protocol analysis plan was to be used. A second analytical complication came from the finding that the non-linearity could have been associated to temporal variations in the ultrasound measurement reproducibility. This observation prompted additional analyses, and the blind rereading of a set of ultrasound examinations confirms that a change in the acquisition and quantitation of ultrasound data could have happened sometime between the 24th and the 36th month of follow up. While the non-linearity observed in MIDAS could not be fully explained, it seems likely that it was associated with an interaction of random and systematic biases in the ultrasound scanning and reading procedures. A correction of the original MIDAS data using factors derived during the rereadings process suggests that the progression of MMax in treated hypertensives may fit a linear model, and that the progression of MMax in treated hypertensives ranges between 0.02 and 0.03mm/yr.

A second major finding was the observation that these trends did not fit with the imbalance in cardiovascular clinical events which were in favor of isradipine (54 vs. 33 in isradipine and HCTZ respectively). This imbalance was mostly confined to one category, i.e., angina pectoris (11 vs. 3 in isradipine and HCTZ respectively). Though the number of events is small, this finding added some concern because of other data reported lately about the potential harm of short acting calcium antagonists (20).

The results and interpretation of MIDAS created a great controversy among investigators, but overall provided a unique framework for designing the forthcoming clinical trials on both hypertension and hypercholesterolemia.

V. CLINICAL TRIALS ON PATIENTS WITH ELEVATED LDL-CHOLESTEROL

Clinical trials directed toward reducing the prevalence of atherosclerosis and its clinical manifestations have been traditionally performed using lipid lowering drugs and dietetic recommendations, and then either counting the reduction in the observed events or quantitating the effects on coronary artery diseases with arteriography. With epidemiological data strongly suggesting the relationship between cholesterol levels and clinical manifestations of atherosclerosis (21), disease prevention has been gaining momentum over disease treatment. Primary prevention of cardiovascular events in patients with elevated LDL-cholesterol is currently the focus of epidemiological and clinical investigations (see previous chapter). As a consequence, several interventional clinical trials were also designed and implemented to test the efficacy of new lipid lowering drugs, i.e, HMGCoA reductase inhibitors, using surrogate endpoints suitable for asymptomatic patients at risk for cardiovascular events.

A. The Pravastatin, Lipid and Atherosclerosis in the Carotid Arteries

The Pravastatin, Lipid and Atherosclerosis in the Carotid Arteries (PLACII) (22,23) was the first interventional controlled clinical trial to be reported in the literature. PLACII tested the antiatherosclerotic effects of lipid lowering using an ultrasonographic outcome measure. PLACII tested the effects of pravastatin, an HMGCoA Reductase Inhibitor, versus placebo on the progression of carotid IMT during a three year follow up study. PLACII was designed to test this hypothesis in a secondary prevention setting. Therefore, selection of the study population aimed at men and women with hypercholesterolemia, a documented history of MI or at least one 0.5 coronary artery stenosis and at least one carotid lesion defined as an IMT larger than 1.3 mm. One hundred and 51 patients (mean age 62.6 years, male 0.85, current smokers 0.12, LDL-cholesterol 165.7 mg/dL, MMax 1.32mm) were randomized to either placebo or pravastatin at an initial dose of 40 mg O.D. In the following 3 months, treatment was adjusted according to the individual patient's response. Specifically, 0.03 of the patients were maintained with 10 mg O.D., 0.24 with 20 mg/day, and 0.73 with 40 mg/day. The PLACII primary and secondary endpoints were the MMax and the TMax, respectively. In PLACII the baseline MMax was 1.32mm, which indicates that patients had ultrasonographic signs of advanced carotid disease. Pravastatin reduced total cholesterol by 0.22, LDL-cholesterol by 0.28, but had no significant effect on HDL-cholesterol. Pravastatin reduced the three year MMax progression rate by 0.12 equal to -0.009mm/yr (p=0.44, non significant). The effect of pravastatin treatment in PLACII was mostly confined to common carotid IMTs (-0.35 or -0.016mm/yr, p<0.03), but no significant changes in progression were observed in the bifurcation and internal carotid arteries or the TMax. PLACII results highlighted a few important points. The yearly progression rate of carotid MMax is low, but the observed precision in estimating this progression is far better than expected. The antiatherosclerotic morphologic effects of lipid lowering may be confined to the earliest stages of plaque development. The efficacy of lipid lowering in decreasing CHD morbidity and mortality may be mediated by morphologic changes of the arterial wall, but other mechanisms may be at least as effective as the reduction in plaque progression.

B. The Asymptomatic Carotid Artery Progression Study

The Asymptomatic Carotid Artery Progression Study (ACAPS) (6,24) was a multicenter interventional controlled clinical trial with a factorial design. ACAPS aimed at testing the morphologic effects of lovastatin, an HMGCoA reductase inhibitors, and warfarin, an antithrombotic agent, in asymptomatic patients with ultrasonographic evidences of carotid atherosclerosis and moderate hypercholesterolemia. Patients were also encouraged to take minidoses of aspirin (81mg O.D.) and postmenopausal women were allowed to use estrogen replacement therapy. Nine hundred and 19 patients were recruited and allocated in 4 treatment groups, i.e., placebo + placebo, lovastatin (10 or 20 or 40mg O.D.) + placebo, placebo + warfarin (1mg O.D.), and lovastatin + warfarin. The ACAPS population mean age was 61.7 year, men were 0.52, had LDL-cholesterol levels of 4.02 mmol/L or 155.6 mg/dL, and the baseline MMax was 1.32 mm. The ACAPS primary endpoint was the MMax. Up to date, ACAPS investigators have extensively reported and published only the effect of lovastatin vs. placebo. ACAPS results show that lovastatin reduced LDL-cholesterol by 0.28, and had minimal effects on HDL-cholesterol and triglycerides. ACAPS was the first trial based on quantitative ultrasound to report the possibility that atherosclerosis can regress. In fact, after a 12 month lag time, the MMax in the following two years of follow up regressed significantly in the lovastatin treated group compared with the control group (-0.009 ± 0.003 vs. 0.006 ± 0.003 mm/yr respectively, $p<0.001$). This direct morphological effect was coupled to a significant benefit on morbid and fatal cardiovascular events (5 vs. 14, $p<0.04$). Because of its sample size and lipid lowering efficacy, ACAPS is certainly a very significant step forward in the understanding of the morphologic effects of HMGCoA reductase inhibitors.

C. The Kuopio Atherosclerotic Plaque Study

The Kuopio Atherosclerotic Plaque Study (KAPS) (6) was a 3 year primary prevention trial of atherosclerosis conducted in the Southern Finnish community of Kuopio. This experiment was relevant because, according to the AHA statistics, Finnish men hold one of the highest CHD mortality rates among industrialized societies (5.8/1000) (25). Secondly, this experiment was conducted by an established team of cardiovascular epidemiologists who have been active for many years, with access to a well characterized population. The design of KAPS focuses on establishing the effects of fixed doses of pravastatin, therefore providing more interpretative ground for a direct morphologic effect of HMGCoA reductase inhibitors on atherosclerosis. Secondly, cigarette smoking status was used as a stratification criteria in order to establish a direct link between nicotine use and treatment efficacy. Four hundred and 24 men (44-65 year, mean 57) were randomized to either a fixed dose of pravastatin (40 mg O.D.) or placebo. KAPS patients were recruited primarily for their hypercholesterolemia (mean baseline LDL-cholesterol: 189.5 mg/dL), without regard to their carotid atherosclerosis status. However, about 10% of the patients had a history of CHD. The study primary ultrasound endpoint was the 3 year changes in CBFMax, which monitors the progression of four, i.e., the far wall of the common and bifurcation bilaterally, of the potential twelve arterial sites as described above. The KAPS baseline carotid IMT was significantly larger than in any reported trial (far wall common carotid IMT: 1.35mm, and far walls common and bifurcation IMT: 1.66mm), suggesting that these patients had advanced and significant carotid atherosclerosis. With a reduction in serum cholesterol similar to PLACII, KAPS showed that, in a three year period, pravastatin achieved a treatment efficacy of 0.45 when compared with placebo for the progression in CBFMax (0.017 ± 0.004 vs 0.031 ± 0.004mm/yr, respectively, $p<0.0005$).

KAPS was the first study to report a significant morphological effect of pravastatin on the progression of carotid IMT, and in addition that smoking significantly affects treatment efficacy. KAPS tends to confirms the PLACII finding that, in patients with more advanced carotid IMT, the maximum treatment efficacy is achieved in the common carotid segments, where IMT is smaller than in the bulb-bifurcation. This seems to reinforce the idea that lipid lowering with HMGCoA Reductase Inhibitors reduces the progression of the earliest stages of atherosclerosis, while may be less effective on more advanced plaques.

D. The Carotid Atherosclerosis Italian Ultrasound Study

The Carotid Atherosclerosis Italian Ultrasound Study (CAIUS) (9,26). CAIUS was the first trial to test the effects of lipid lowering on the progression of carotid intima-media thickness in 305 asymptomatic men and women with moderate hypercholesterolemia, at least one carotid lesion (1.3<TMax<3.5mm), and cardiovascular asymptomatic status. CAIUS, contrary to KAPS is relevant because it studied the effect of fixed doses of pravastatin on the progression of atherosclerosis in a population known to have lower cholesterol levels, and where CHD mortality is less prevalent (men 3.4/1000, women

1.5/1000) (25). Therefore, this trial provided an experimental setting in which the potential direct morphological benefits of HMGCoA reductase inhibitors could be studied without the main interference of extreme hypercholesterolemia and other factors which may be responsible for increased mortality. The 305 CAIUS patients were on average 55 years old, 0.53 male, mean LDL were 4.68mmol/L, and HDL=1.37mmol/L. Patients were assigned to pravastatin (40mg O.D., n.151) or placebo (n.154). The carotid MMax was chosen as the primary endpoint, and the difference between the two treatment 3 year progression slopes as the primary outcome measure. Five serious cardiovascular events (1 fatal MI) and 7 drop-outs for cancer were registered. In the pravastatin group, LDL decreased -0.22 after 3 months vs. -0.01 in the placebo group, and remained substantially stable afterward (-0.23 vs. +0.01 at 36 months, respectively). Progression of the MMax was 0.009 ± 0.0027, and -0.0043 ± 0.0028 mm/yr ($p<0.0007$) in the placebo and pravastatin groups, respectively. IMT progression slopes diverged after 6 months of treatment with the placebo group progressing steadily throughout the duration of the study, and the pravastatin group lagging around the zero line, i.e., no progression/regression.

The CAIUS findings show that pravastatin stops the progression of carotid IMT in asymptomatic, moderately hypercholesterolemic men and women. This finding extends the beneficial effects of cholesterol lowering to the primary prevention of atherosclerosis in a population with relatively low cardiovascular event rates and suggests that this benefit is mediated by specific morphological effects on early stages of plaque development. These findings are important because the balanced design of CAIUS, i.e., an appropriate sample size and an optimal representation of women, adds significantly to the current view that an important quota of the benefits achieved through lipid lowering with HMGCoA reductase inhibitors may be mediated by a direct action on the plaque.

VI. OTHER ONGOING CLINICAL TRIALS

A significant number of new clinical trials to test the effects of blood pressure lowering drugs were initiated after the presentations of the design and some baseline information from MIDAS. With the exception of one trial testing the effects of verapamil, the post-MIDAS era includes trials aimed at testing the morphologic effects of the new generation of calcium antagonists, which seemed to have better pharmacodynamics, i.e., amlodipine (Prospective Randomized Evaluation of the Vascular Effects of Norvasc Trial,

PREVENT), and possibly antioxidant activities, i.e., lacidipine, α-blockers, i.e., doxazosin (Doxazosin Atherosclerosis Progression Study in Hypertensives in the Netherlands, DAPHNE), and ACE-inhibitors, i.e., perindropil, ramipril (Prevention of Atherosclerosis with Ramipril Therapy, PART; Study to Evaluate Carotid Ultrasound Changes with Ramipril and Vitamin E, SECURE), and fosinopril.

A. The Verapamil Hypertension Atherosclerosis Study

Though results of the Verapamil Hypertension Atherosclerosis Study (VHAS) (27) are not available yet, this clinical trial is important because it was one of the first clinical trial on hypertension initiated in Europe using an ultrasound endpoint.

VHAS is a multicenter investigation which involves 80 Italian hypertension clinics, and monitors the clinical effects of verapamil SR (240 mg O.D.), a calcium antagonist, and chlorthalidone (25 mg O.D.), a diuretic, in 1,450 males and females (40 to 65 years old) with primary hypertension. A subgroup of 500 subjects was randomly selected to be prospectively examined with B-mode ultrasound imaging. In this subgroup of patients, the investigators will attempt to determine the efficacy of the two treatment regimens in slowing the progression of ultrasonically detected and monitored carotid plaques.

It is unsure whether the ultrasound protocol used in this trial meets the standard criteria used in other studies. Some concerns point to the use of ultrasound instrumentation with different frequencies, one of the factors that makes inter laboratory standardization difficult. However, findings from this trial are important especially after questions were raised by the results of MIDAS and other metanalytical works.

B. The Perindopril Regression of Vascular Thickening European Community Trial

The Perindopril Regression of Vascular Thickening European Community Trial (PROTECT) (28) is a prospective multicenter clinical trial involving 16 Medical Centers in 9 European countries including Austria, Belgium, France, Germany, Italy, the Netherlands, Spain, Switzerland, and the United Kingdom. The PROTECT primary objective is to determine the efficacy of perindopril, an ACE-inhibitor, and HCTZ, a diuretic, in controlling the progression of common carotid IMT over a two year period of treatment. Baseline and the two year changes in the common carotid IMT of a minimum of 800 asymptomatic patients with high blood pressure will be assessed with B-mode ultrasound imaging. Eligible patients have an age between 35 and 55 years, must have a sitting systolic blood pressure in the range of 95-110 mmHg after a 4 week placebo wash out trial, and a minimum common carotid IMT of 0.8mm. The PROTECT patients will be also examined to determine femoral atherosclerosis, left ventricular hypertrophy, ambulatory blood pressure and electrocardiographic changes.

While a detailed description of the trial design and a specific operational definition of the ultrasound endpoints are not available at this time, it seems that, based on information available from other trials and the theoretical considerations discussed above, a 2 year follow up may fall short of showing the real morphological effects of perindropil on IMT. However, combined with the results of other trials on different ACE-inhibitors, and because of the significant number of patients being recruited, the forthcoming findings of PROTECT will add important insights into the efficacy of ACE-inhibitors on vascular protection.

C. The European Lacidipine Study on Atherosclerosis

The European Lacidipine Study on Atherosclerosis (ELSA) (29) will compare the effects of lacidipine with those of the β-blocker atenolol in preventing the progression of vascular injuries. ELSA is a 4-year follow-up, multi-national, multicenter clinical trial. A cohort of about 2,300 hypertensive patients (95 mmHg≤diastolic blood pressure≤115 mmHg, systolic blood pressure≤210 mmHg) have been recruited in 230 European clinical centers during an 18 month period. The clinical centers are responsible for managing the patients' treatment and periodic medical routines. Twenty three highly specialized referral centers, located in major academic medical centers in 7 European countries including France, Germany, Greece, Italy, Spain, Sweden, and the United Kingdom, will provide expertise in quantitative vascular and cardiac ultrasonography and ambulatory blood pressure monitoring.   The patients were randomized into two treatment arms (experimental: lacidipine , 4-6 mg O.D.; control: atenolol, 50-100 mg O.D.). Refractory patients in both groups will be controlled with open label HCTZ (12.5-25 mg)

The study primary objective is to determine the efficacy of lacidipine and atenolol in slowing the progression of carotid IMT. The study primary hypothesis is that lacidipine, while reducing blood pressure comparably to β-blockers and the associated hemodynamic actions on the arterial wall, offers superior vascular protection due to specific effects on endothelial and smooth muscle cells, matrix production, and its antioxidant properties. This hypothesis will be tested using carotid IMT as a surrogate measurements of hypertension related vascular damage. Quantitative B-mode ultrasound will be administered annually for up to 4 years, and for each patient the common and bifurcation mean maximum IMT (CBMax) slope of progression will be calculated. The primary endpoint for the study is the group difference in the 4 year progression of CBMax.

In lieu of the recent debate surrounding the safety of calcium antagonists in patients at risk of cardiac ischemia, because of the size of the population studied and the extensive use of powerful diagnostic tests, ELSA is going to have a major impact in the future use of calcium antagonists and β-blockers in the care of hypertension. Secondly, being the single largest clinical trial using an interlaboratory standardized B-mode ultrasound protocol, ELSA will provide a unique database which will probably define the future applicability and application of this technique for testing hypotheses with surrogate endpoints.

D. The Plaque Hypertension Lipid Lowering Italian Study

The Plaque Hypertension Lipid Lowering Italian Study (PHYLLIS) (30) is an innovative clinical trial in which, for the first time, investigators will test whether an additive protective effect on atherosclerosis progression can be achieved with a combination of treatments to control hypertension and to reduce LDL-cholesterol levels. Specifically, PHYLLIS is a multicenter clinical trial aimed at testing the morphologic effects of pravastatin, a HMGCoA reductase inhibitor, and fosinopril, an ACE-inhibitor, on the progression of carotid atherosclerosis in asymptomatic hypercholesterolemics with moderate primary hypertension. This hypothesis will be tested using a factorial design with four pharmacological treatments, including placebo + HCTZ (25mg O.D.), pravastatin (40mg O.D.) + HCTZ, placebo + fosinopril (20mg O.D.), and pravastatin + fosinopril. Atenolol will be used open label, if hypertension is not adequately controlled by the experimental treatments. After a 4-6 weeks run in period, 800 eligible patients (diastolic blood pressure 95-115 mmHg, LDL-cholesterol 160-200 mg/dL, and ultrasonographic evidences of early carotid atherosclerosis, i.e., 1.3<IMT<3.5mm) will be randomized into one of the four treatment groups. The trial primary outcome measure is the common carotid and bifurcation mean maximum IMT (CBMax), while the primary endpoint is the 3 year difference in the progression of CBMax. Carotid IMT progressions will be estimated with quantitative B-mode ultrasound imaging performed annually for three years. The primary hypothesis is that the combination of pravastatin plus fosinopril provides higher protection than a less effective lipid lowering strategy (i.e., low fat diet), and/or HCTZ.

The PHYLLIS hypothesis is certainly an important one. In fact, while no data are available on the efficacy of combination treatments, the true target for primary prevention intervention is mostly on patients with associated risk factors for accelerated atherosclerosis. Furthermore, it seems that the association of hypertension and hypercholesterolemia is highly prevalent, while it goes often unrecognized until it is too late.

VII. SIGNIFICANCE AND LIMITATIONS OF INTERVENTIONAL CLINICAL TRIALS

The most effective treatment aimed at reducing LDL-cholesterol levels, i.e. , HMG CoA reductase inhibition, has shown to reduce total and/or cardiovascular mortality in large clinical trials. In different experimental settings, though smaller in size, these beneficial effects on morbidity and mortality have been accompanied by a slow decrease of the carotid IMT progression. On the contrary, in at least one study on hypertension, i.e. , MIDAS, the lack of effects on carotid IMT progression was observed concomitantly to an increase of cardiovascular events. These observations, together with a cohort of information derived from epidemiologic studies, have increased the value of this technique which in addition offers good sensitivity, acceptable reproducibility, low costs and last but not least, total noninvasivity. However, new questions arise as well. In fact, while atherosclerosis is an arterial wall phenomenon, the resulting clinical event is many times associated with an acute reduction of the arterial lumen. At this regard, very limited information exists linking the distributions and changes of IMT to lumen dimensions. Some reports have suggested that this relationship is not constant, but varies according to the arterial segment. For example, it seems that while changes in IMT and lumen go in the same direction in the distal common carotid artery, the relation inverts in the proximal internal carotid artery. If this proves true, the finding may have some impact on the current interpretation of clinical trial results. In addition, it may have an effect in choosing ultrasound endpoints and especially on the current practice to average several arterial segments which certainly have different biological characteristics, and may also have a different pathobiology.

A second set of questions refers to the clinical relevance of being able to detect and monitor in large group of patient microscopic changes at the level of the arterial wall. The first implication is whether these findings can be extrapolated to the individual patients. Sophisticated statistical analyses seem to suggest that B-mode ultrasound is sensitive enough to detect cross sectional differences in IMT among individual patients (10). However, at present the sensitivity of the technique does not allow to identify different rates of progression in individual patients unless the follow up is extended over several years and includes numerous visits. The second implication is whether it is possible, on an individual patient basis, to use B-mode ultrasound criteria to extrapolate the status of coronary artery disease and/or to have any chance to predict an impending clinical event. At this time there is no evidence that this could be accomplished on an individual basis. However, it needs to be underlined that the above question cannot be answered by any single technique either noninvasive or invasive. Certainly, today's diagnostic armamentarium includes techniques which, if rationally integrated, offer ample ground for identifying patients at risk and treating them more efficiently and cost-effectively than in the past.

VIII. SUMMARY

B-mode ultrasound imaging protocols are being used in large multinational-multicenter controlled clinical trials to test the morphologic effects of treatments directed toward reducing cardiovascular risk. Information derived from multiple applications of this technique shows that B-mode ultrasound is reliable and effective in detecting small changes occurring in the arterial wall as a consequence of atherogenic factors or their pharmacological control.

Acknowledgments

Our gratitude goes to Prof. Alessandro Ventura, University of Perugia, Italy, Dr. Mariarita Pignatelli, Bowman Gray School of Medicine, USA, Dr. Fabrizio Veglia, San Raffaele Scientific Institute, Milan, Italy, and Mr. Michael Hennig, Munich Technical University, Germany. This work was supported in part by grants from the following companies: Bristol-Myers Squibb S.p.A, Italy; Boehringer Ingelheim, Germany; Glaxo-Wellcome S.p.A., Italy; Menarini Industrie Farmaceutiche Riunite, Italy; Sandoz Research Institute, and Vasocor Inc., U.S.A..

References

1. Shepherd J, Cobbe SM, Ford I et al. for the West of Scotland Coronary Prevention Study Group. Prevention of Coronary Heart Disease With Pravastatin in Men With Hypercholesterolemia. N Engl J Med 1995; 333:1301-7
2. Scandinavian Simvastatin Survival Study Group. Baseline Serum Cholesterol and Treatment Effect in the Scandinavian Simvastatin Survival Study (4S). Lancet 1995; 345:1274-1275
3. Sacks FM, Pfeffer MA, Moye LA et al. for the Cholesterol and Recurrent Events Trial Investigators: The Effects of Pravastatin on Coronary Events After Myocardial Infarction in Patients with Average Cholesterol Levels. N Engl J Med 1996; 335:1001-9
4. Mercuri M: Noninvasive Imaging Protocols to Detect and Monitor Carotid Atherosclerosis Progression. American Journal of Hypertension 1994; 7:23S-29S
5. Berglund GL: Minisymposium: Ultrasound in Clinical Trials of Atherosclerosis. Introduction. Journal of Internal Medicine 1994; 236: 551-553
6. Furberg CD, Adams HP Jr, Applegate WB et al. for the Asymptomatic Carotid Artery Progression Study (ACAPS) Research Group. Effects of Lovastatin on Early Carotid Atherosclerosis and Cardiovascular Events. Circulation 1994; 90:1676-1687
7. Salonen R, Nyyssönen K, Porkkala E et al.: Kuopio Atherosclerosis Prevention Study (KAPS). A Population-Based Primary Prevention Trial of the Effect of LDL Lowering on Atherosclerotic Progression in Carotid and Femoral Arteries. Circulation 1995; 92(7): 1758-1764
8. Borhani NO, Mercuri M, Borhani PA et al.: Final Outcome of the Multicenter Isradipine Diuretic Atherosclerosis Study (MIDAS). A Randomized Controlled Trial. JAMA 1996; 276:785-791
9. Mercuri M, Bond MG, Sirtori CR et al.: Pravastatin Reduces Carotid Intima media Thickness Progression in an Asymptomatic Hypercholesterolemic Mediterranean population. The Carotid Atherosclerosis Italian Ultrasound Study. Am J Med 1996; 101:627-634
10. Espeland MA, Craven TE, Riley WA et al. For the Asymptomatic Carotid Artery progression Study: Reliability of Longitudinal Ultrasonographic Measurements of Carotid Intimal-Medial Thickness. Stroke 1996; 27:480-485
11. Chobanian AV: The 1989 Corcoran Lecture: Adaptation and Maladptive Responses of the Arterial Wall to Hypertension. Hypertension 1990;1 5:666-674
12. MacMahon SW, Cutler JA, Furberg CD, Payne GH: The Effects of Drug Treatment for Hypertension on Morbidity and Mortality from cardiovascular Disease: A Review of Randomized Controlled Trials. Prog Cardiovasc Dis 1986; 29(suppl. 1):99-118
13. Collins R, Peto R, MacMahon S: Blood Pressure, Stroke, and Coronary Hearth Disease, part II: Short Term Reduction in Blood Pressure, Overview of randomized Drug Trials in Their Epidemiological Context. Lancet 1990; 335:827-838
14. Weinstein DB, Heider JC: Antiatherogenic Properties of calcium Antagonists. Am J cardiol 1987; 59:163B-172B
15. Bond MG, Purvis C, Mercuri M: Antiatherogenic Properties of calcium Antagonists. J Cardiovasc Pharmacol 1991; 17(suppl. 4):87-93
16. Lichtlen PR, Hugenholtz PG, Rafflenbeul W et al.: Retardation of Angiographic Progression of Coronary Artery Disease by Nifedipine. Results of the International Nifedipine Trial on Anti-atherosclerotic Therapy (INTACT). Lancet 1990; 335:1109-1113
17. Waters D, Lespérance J, Francetich M et al.: A Controlled Clinical trial to Assess the Effect of a Calcium Channel Blocker on the Progression of Coronary Atherosclerosis. Circulation 1990;82:1940-1953
18. Furberg CD, Byington RP, Craven TE. Lessons learned from clinical trials with ultrasound endpoints. J Int Med 1994; 236:575-80.
19. Mercuri M, Bond MG, Nichols FT, et al.: Baseline Reproducibility of B-mode Ultrasound Imaging Measurements of Carotid Intima Media Thickness: The Multicenter Isradipine Diuretic Atherosclerosis Study (MIDAS). J Cardiovascular Diagnosis and Procedures 1993; 11:241-255
20. Chobanian AV: Calcium Channel Blockers. Lessons Learned from MIDAS and Other Clinical Trials. JAMA 1996; 276:829-830
21. Holme I, Enger SC, Helgeland A, et al.: Risk Factors and Raised Atherosclerotic Lesions in Coronary and Cerebral Arteries. Arteriosclerosis 1981; 1:250-256
22. Crouse JR, Byington RP, Bond MG, et al.: Pravastatin, lipids and atherosclerosis in the carotid arteries: design features of a clinical trial with carotid atherosclerosis outcome. Control Clin Trials 1992; 13:495-506.
23. Crouse JR III, Byington RP, Bond MG, et al.: Pravastatin, Lipids, and Atherosclerosis in the Carotid Arteries (PLACII). American Journal of Cardiology 1995; 75:455-459
24. The ACAPS Group: Rationale and Design for the Asymptomatic Carotid Artery Plaque Study (ACAPS). Control Clin Trials 1992; 13:293-314

25. American Heart Association: Heart and Stroke Facts: 1996 Statistical Supplement. Dallas, TX, 1996, p. 8.
26. Sirtori CR, Bianchi G, Bond MG, et al.: Pravastatin Intervention Trial on Carotid Artery Atherosclerosis in Patients With Mild Hypercholesterolemia: The CAIUS Study. International Journal of Cardiac Imaging 1995; 11(Suppl 2):119-124
27. Zanchetti A, Magnani B, Dal Palú C for the VHAS Group: Atherosclerosis and calcium Antagonists: The VHAS. J Human Hypertension 1992; 6(suppl. 2):S45-S48
28. Ludwig M, Stumpe KO, Heagerty AM et al. For the PROTECT Group: Vascular Thickness in Hypertension: The Perindopril Regression of Vascular Thickening European Community Trial (PROTECT). J Hypertension 1993; 11(suppl. 5):S316-S317
29. Zanchetti A: Calcium Antagonists in Atherosclerosis and Assessment of their Effect in Clinical Trials: The European Lacidipine Study on Atherosclerosis (ELSA). JAMA Southeast Asia 1994; 10:44-47
30. The PHYLLIS Group: Plaque Hypertension Lipid-Lowering Italian Study (PHYLLIS): A Protocol for Non-invasive Evaluation of Carotid Atherosclerosis in Hypercholesterolemic Hypertensive Subjects. J Hypertension 1993; 11(suppl. 5);S314-S315

SECTION III

PERSPECTIVES IN ULTRASOUND IMAGING

THE ROLE OF MECHANICS IN VASCULAR BIOLOGY

Krishnan B. Chandran, D.Sc. and Michael J. Vonesh, Ph.D.

*University of Iowa, Biomedical Engineering, Iowa City, Iowa;
Northwestern University, Chicago, Illinois U.S.A.*

Contents

I. INTRODUCTION:

Intrinsic material properties of arterial tissue play an important role in vascular physiology. Arterial material properties are thought to influence: passive mechanical behavior of large arteries (1-3), vessel reactivity to neural, humoral and hemodynamic stimuli (4,5), mass transport within the arterial wall (5-7), blood flow through an arterial segment (6, 8, 9), evolution and influence of atherosclerotic and hypertensive disease (10-14), stress distribution within the arterial wall (15-20), and arterial response to therapeutic intervention (21-23). The ability to accurately determine the material properties of the arterial wall has wide ranging clinical, engineering, and basic science implications.

Various pathophysiological conditions alter the material properties of arterial tissue, the most clinically relevant being atherosclerosis and hypertension-induced arteriosclerosis. Atherosclerosis is a disease of the arterial wall characterized by the subendothelial accumulation of lipid and necrotic debris, smooth muscle cell (SMC) proliferation, and connective tissue synthesis. In most vascular beds, this process gradually progresses toward the formation of heterogeneous occlusive lesions (or plaques), and is accompanied by compensatory remodeling of arterial wall morphology (24,25). Although atherosclerosis is the principal cause of death in Western countries, the etiology of atherosclerosis is poorly understood (26). Most hypotheses forwarded to explain atherosclerosis assert that atherogenesis is a multifactorial disease process in which hemodynamic, genetic, behavioral, and biochemical risk factors are thought to play a role (6,26,27). Clinical manifestations of atherosclerosis are attributable to: inhibition of normal blood flow, compromised vascular reactivity, and spontaneous rupture of advanced atherosclerotic lesions (28). Previous work has demonstrated that atherosclerosis alters the composition and mechanical properties of arterial tissue (29-31). Similarly, chronic hypertension is associated with alterations of the arterial wall (e.g., diffuse fibrosis and intimal thickening) that are also known to change the fundamental mechanical behavior of arterial tissue (32,33).

Biomechanical analysis techniques provide a means of quantifying the normal behavior of vascular tissue, and determining the extent and physiological significance of vascular disease. The study of vascular mechanical behavior has been the subject of scientific study for over 200 years. Historical developments in biomechanics, including those relating to circulation and vascular mechanics, are summarized in (34).

Contributions to the description of human circulation by William Harvey in 1615, and to the formulation of the pressure pulse wave propagation and hydrodynamics theories of circulation by Korteweg, Lamb, Frank, and Womersley are noteworthy. This area remains one of active investigation. Recent progress in computationally intensive numerical analysis techniques, such as finite element analysis, together with advances in the three-dimensional reconstruction of ultrasound imaging data, may be exploited to generate highly accurate mechanical analyses of in-vivo vascular segments under normal and pathological conditions.

Continued development of biomechanical analysis techniques are likely to enhance our understanding of both vascular mechanical behavior and basic vascular physiology. In the clinical arena, accurate identification of the functional significance of cardiovascular disease may facilitate decisions to institute medical countermeasures (i.e., dietary, behavioral, or pharmacological), to select therapeutic interventions optimized to the target lesion, or to identify candidates for surgical recannulation. Vascular mechanical parameters may additionally provide useful end points in evaluating the results of a prescribed therapy, and have the potential to allow on-going or periodic evaluation of patients subjected to various interventions. In the field of biomedical engineering, design of vascular prostheses, catheter-based interventional devices (e.g., stents, angioplasty, atherectomy, roto-ablation), and circulatory assist devices benefit from vascular mechanics knowledge. Lastly, it is becoming increasingly apparent that biomechanical factors act as important stimuli to various endothelial signal transduction pathways (35,36) .

In this chapter, a brief review of the measurement and analysis techniques used in the determination of mechanical properties of vascular segments is discussed, along with potential applications of ultrasound.

II.   MECHANICAL ANALYSIS OF VASCULAR SEGMENTS

Numerous attempts have been reported to describe the rheological behavior (stress-strain relationship) of blood vessels. An overview of our understanding of the mechanics of blood vessels is included below, pertinent to our goal of analyzing vascular reactivity in the normal and diseased states. Hayashi (33) has presented a succinct review of the classical 0.vascular mechanics literature, whereas Simon et al. (7) have reviewed the use of finite element models in describing the rheology of blood vessel segments.

A. Anatomy of the Arterial Wall

The normal arterial wall is an in homogeneous composite material consisting of three distinct layers. The inner most layer of the arterial wall, the intima, consists of a layer of endothelial cells overlying a thin substrate containing elastin. The function of the endothelial cells is to provide a smooth, non-thrombogenic interface between the blood and the intramural structural components of the wall. Additionally, the endothelial cells play a role in regulating mass transport between the bloodstream and intramural tissues (e.g., they are selectively permeable to water, electrolytes, sugars and other metabolites), and are also thought to incorporate a variety of receptor apparati (i.e., electrolyte channels, adhesion molecules) sensitive to both chemical (e.g., adenosine triphosphate, nitrous oxide, prostacylin) and mechanical (e.g., stretch, shear, shear gradient) stimuli. The internal elastic lamina separates the intima from the middle layer, the media. The media consists of varying proportions of elastin, collagen, and vascular smooth muscle. Elastin is present in all the vessels except the capillaries and venules, and is highly distensible. Collagen fibers form a dense network in the media and are much stiffer than the elastin (approximately 300 times; (37)). The anatomical configuration of the collagen fibers is such that their contribution to the structural support of the artery is related to transmural pressure. As transmural pressure increases, vessel distension increases and the degree of inherent slackness exhibited by collagen fibers decreases. This process results in recruitment of collagen fibers to assume a greater share of supporting hoop stresses in the arterial wall, thus contributing to an increase in the structural rigidity of the vessel. Together, the elastin and collagen fibers maintain a residual passive tension on the artery that counteracts the transmural pressure acting on the intimal surface. The remaining component of the media, vascular smooth muscle, contributes physiologically controlled vasoactive tone to the arterial wall. Medial smooth muscle plays an active part in regulating the vascular resistance to flow and controlling the distribution of blood between various compartments of the body. The external elastic lamina separates the media from the outer layer of the vessel wall, the adventitia. The adventitia contains connective tissue that merges with the surrounding tissue, tethering the vessel in-situ. Refer to Figure 1a. In atherosclerosis, both the composition and structure of the afflicted artery changes from the normal state. Depending upon the stage of disease progression, the composition of the diseased artery generally includes increased smooth muscle cells (SMC), fibrosclerotic tissue, and calcification. The cross-sectional shape of the lumen in most vessels is markedly eccentric, however concentric lesion do occur (25). Additionally, in most arterial beds compensatory enlargement of the arterial structure occurs concurrently with atherosclerotic plaque formation. This process involves both thinning of the medial tissue and enlargement of total arterial area in an attempt to preserve residual lumen area. Compensatory remodeling is limited, however, and progressive increases in plaque mass can eventually overtake the ability of the artery to remodel. Once the compensatory reserve is exhausted, plaque encroachment into the lumen, and clinical manifestations, may begin. (24). More recent studies indicate that a decrease in internal elastic lamina area, consistent with local shrinkage of the artery, may be observed in atherosclerotic arteries (38). Wall shrinkage is suggested as a form of arterial remodeling that aggravates rather than alleviates the flow obstruction presented by the atherosclerotic plaque. See Figure 1b.

Hypertension is generally accompanied by fibrosclerotic hyperplasia often resulting in diffuse thickening of the intimal layer of the arteries, with concomitant changes in arterial material properties. The elevated blood pressure results in an increase in the vessel diameter and reduced vascular compliance. These effects, however, are not due to the stretching of the artery alone, but also due to: intrinsic alterations of the arterial walls (39), or excessive smooth muscle tone (14). The delineation of vascular material property alterations due to the concomitant effect of hypertension, aging, and atherosclerosis poses a difficult challenge.

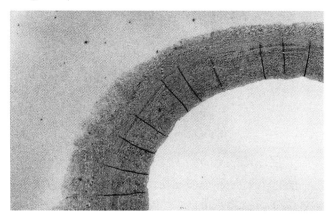

Figure 1a.   Anatomy of normal arterial wall.

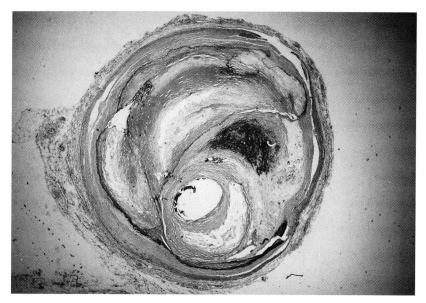

Figure 1b.   Anatomy of atherosclerotic arterial wall.

B.   Basic Definitions and Assumptions Used in Vascular Mechanics

Mechanical studies of vascular tissue are largely derived from methods used to evaluate conventional engineering materials. Due to the obvious differences in the nature of these materials, application of conventional approaches to study biological tissues often requires certain simplifying assumptions and experimental constraints. To provide all readers with a common point of reference, a brief summary of pertinent terminology, assumptions, and experimental considerations is provided.

Rheology The study of deformation and flow of material due to forces acting on the same.

Test Specimen Sample of vascular tissue subjected to mechanical analysis. Ex-vivo test specimens commonly take the form of isolated strips, rings, patches, or tubular segments. In-vivo test specimens might be considered a localized region of a specific blood vessel.

Stress (σ) Stress is defined as the force per unit cross-sectional area of a specimen under consideration. In engineering practice, the forces are resolved into components perpendicular and tangential to the cross-sectional area. Thus stresses are defined as normal (perpendicular to the cross-sectional area) and shear (tangential to the area) stresses.

Strain (ϵ) Strain is defined as the magnitude of deformation experienced by a specimen, in response to application of force, normalized to an appropriate initial dimension. Typically, an axial strain is the ratio of change in length of a specimen along the axis over the initial unstressed length.

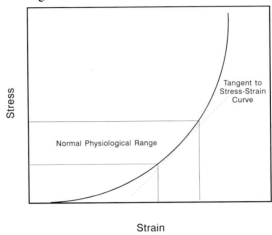

Figure 2. A schematic of the circumferential stress vs. internal radius plot for a blood vessel.

Elasticity The ability of a test specimen to return to its original, undeformed shape upon removal of an applied load is known as elasticity. An ideal elastic solid deforms instantly when stressed, and returns instantly to its original dimensions when stress is removed. Elastic strain energy stored in the material during stressing is completely recoverable (without loss) upon removal of the stress. A *linear elastic material* is said to obey Hooke's law. This implies that stress and strain are directly related, and the ratio of stress to strain (i.e., the slope of this function) is defined as the elastic (or Young's) modulus. The elastic modulus represents the inherent stiffness of the material. Most common engineering materials exhibit a linear stress-strain relationship within limits of deformation for practical applications. The elastic modulus for rubber is about 4×10^7 dynes/cm^2, and for structural steel, it is 2×10^{12} dynes/cm^2. The elastic modulus for arteries is of the order of $1 - 20 \times 10^6$ dynes/cm^2. Most biological soft tissues, including the blood vessel wall, exhibit a non-linear stress-strain relationship within the range of physiological loading. At lower transmural pressures, the mechanical behavior of the vessel is primarily governed by elastin and smooth muscle. At higher pressures, collagen fibers dominate the mechanical behavior and hence the vessel becomes stiffer. Because elastin and smooth muscle are much more compliant than collagen, the relationship between stress and strain becomes non-linear. A typical plot of stress as a function of internal radius for a vessel, as shown in Figure 2, demonstrates this non-linear relationship. To simplify biomechanical analysis, a linear stress-strain relationship is often assumed for short increments in loading (a step-wise linear approach). It is customary to define the tangent to the non-linear stress-strain relationship, over small increments in strain, as the incremental elastic modulus(E_{inc}).   Plotting the incremental elastic modulus as a function of transmural pressure is a useful method of characterizing mechanical behavior of vascular tissue.

The incremental elastic modulus (E_{inc}) is defined as the tangent to the non-linear stress vs.strain relationship. In the normal physiological range (i.e., pressures between 80 mm Hg and 120 mm Hg), the stress-strain relationship is often approximated as being linear.

Poisson's Ratio (μ) Elongation of a test specimen along one direction ordinarily results in contraction in the other two directions or vice versa. The ratio of the transverse (or lateral) contracting strain to the longitudinal elongating strain is defined as the Poisson's ratio. Poisson's ratio is an inherent material property. For ideal, incompressible materials μ = 0.5.

Constitutive Relationship The constitutive relationship, or material law, defines a material's deformation (strain) in response to an applied stress. The mechanical behavior of any material is characterized by its constitutive relationship.

Incompressibility Characteristic of a material whose volume remains constant when subjected to a hydrostatic pressure. The arterial wall has been demonstrated to be nearly incompressible (40,41).

Homogeneity Homogeneity of material properties implies that mechanical behavior is uniform throughout the tissue (i.e., independent of location).   It is often sufficient to treat the vessel wall as homogeneous (within the physiological range of loading) in order to analyze the rheological behavior of normal arteries or to differentiate the effects of diseased states on the same. Utilization of this assumption to facilitate analysis of atherosclerotic arterial tissue, however, is a gross over simplification.

Isotropy If a material property is independent of direction, or, equivalently, that the material properties are uniform in all directions, it is said to be isotropic. A simplifying assumption in many biomechanical analysis is that the arterial vessel wall is isotropic. Weizsacker and Pinto (42) as well as Dobrin (43) suggest that the arterial wall can be treated as isotropic within the physiological range of deformation, however, numerous studies have shown that the vessels exhibit anisotropic behavior.

Orthotropy A material is defined as orthotropic or transversely isotropic if the material properties are different in mutually orthogonal (perpendicular) directions. In a cylindrically defined coordinate system, as is often used in vascular mechanics, the radial, circumferential, and axial (longitudinal) directions are mutually orthogonal. Patel et al. (44,45), for example, demonstrated that the elastic modulus in the circumferential direction was larger than that in the radial direction with the magnitude in the axial direction being the largest. They attributed the largest modulus in the axial direction to the tethering of the vessels longitudinally. Similar results have also been reported in more recent studies (46,47). However, other studies have reported that the elastic modulus in the circumferential direction is stiffer than in the axial direction (48,49) . Tanaka and Fung (50) showed that the elastic modulus in the longitudinal direction is stiffer than in the circumferential direction for the canine thoracic aorta and vice versa in the iliac and femoral arteries. Hayashi (33) attributes these contradicting results to variations in experimental methods, species differences as well as in the arterial sites investigated.

Vascular Compliance Compliance of a vascular segment is defined as the ratio of volumetric strain (increment in vessel wall volume to the original volume) to increment in pressure. It can also be expressed as increase in radius to the initial radius for a given increase in pressure. Vascular compliance tends to decrease with age, and also in the presence of hypertension and atherosclerosis.

Experimental Considerations

The passive elastic properties of the individual components of the vessel wall have been compared with those of common engineering materials (37). Uniaxial and biaxial tensile tests on flat strips extracted from arterial specimens (51-53), and atherosclerotic plaques (30,31,54,55) have also been attempted. Although much basic knowledge has been gained through mechanical testing of isolated arterial tissue strips, a better understanding of the mechanical behavior of blood vessels is perhaps obtained through the study of the force-deformation characteristics (pressure-diameter relationship) of intact vessels. Mechanical testing of intact blood vessels typically involves subjecting vascular specimens to a range of transmural pressures while measuring concurrent changes in arterial diameter (internal, external) and/or wall thickness.   Theories of elasticity or viscoelasticity can then be invoked to analyze the material properties of the vessels.

In performing in-vitro experiments of this sort, the physiological environment of ionic content, moisture, temperature and other variables must be comparable to that experienced by the blood vessels in situ. Since the blood vessels are tethered along the axial direction in situ, the length can decrease by about 40 percent once the blood vessel is excised. This must be accounted for while performing the in-vitro biomechanical testing. Additionally, in-vitro testing of vascular tissue should be preceded by cyclic loading over the physiological range to precondition the arterial tissue. It is necessary to perform the loading and unloading cycle a number of times before the stress-strain results are repeatable(34, 56). Experimental stresses imposed upon the arterial tissue may be either static or dynamic, depending on the nature of the investigation. In static testing, sufficient time (generally > 2 minutes) must elapse for the tissue to achieve a steady state (equilibrium) level of strain in response to an applied load (57).

Measurable variables for the study of intact arterial specimens include intraluminal pressure, arterial diameter, wall thickness, and length.   It is important   that the measurement approaches employed do not adversely influence the behavior of the tissue being measured. Pressure is readily obtained with standard physiological transducers, however, measurements of arterial geometry are more difficult. Megerman et al. (58) specify that measurement of the geometrical variables must be reproducible, applicable over a wide range of pressures, mechanically unrestrictive, and, preferably, non-invasive to accurately describe the elastic properties of arterial tissue. Given the morphological variability of atherosclerosis, measurement and analysis techniques should also allow *regional* characterization of arterial tissue behavior.   Most conventional approaches (8,58,60) are unable to comply with these requirements because geometrical measurements are made at a localized site within the vessel. These measurements, particularly in disease states may not be representative of the entire segment. Analysis based on these techniques thus yield a global value of elasticity or stiffness characterizing the average behavior of the entire vessel segment.

C.   Conventional Approaches to Describe the Vascular Mechanical Behavior

1. Static Pressure, Thin-Walled Cylinder Approach

In determining inherent material properties (e.g., elasticity) from the pressure-radius relationship, for example, it is often assumed that the vessel segment geometry is circularly cylindrical and that it is composed of a homogeneous, isotropic, incompressible Hookean (linearly elastic) material. If the vessel wall thickness, h, is sufficiently small compared to the vessel radius, R (h/R $\ll$ 0.1),the vessel can be assumed to be a thin-walled cylindrical pressure vessel.   In that case, the relationship between the circumferential stress, σ_θ, and circumferential strain, ϵ_θ, can be expressed as (61):

$$\sigma_\theta = \frac{pR}{h},\qquad (1)$$

and

$$\epsilon_\theta = \frac{\Delta R}{R},\qquad (2)$$

where p is the transmural pressure and ΔR is the increment in the internal radius of the vessel. This situation is depicted in Figure 3a. The circumferential elastic modulus (E_θ) of the material comprising the vessel wall is given by the relationship:

$$E_\theta = \frac{\sigma_\theta}{\epsilon_\theta} = \frac{pR^2}{h\Delta R}.\qquad (3)$$

Thus, if the vessel wall can be classified as a thin-walled pressure vessel and the wall material is assumed to be linearly elastic (i.e., with a constant elastic modulus, E, computed as the ratio of the stress and strain), the above relationship can be employed to estimate the elastic properties in normal vascular segments.

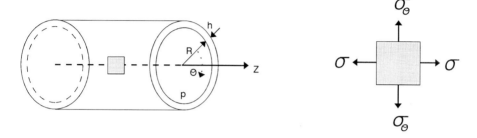

Figure 3a. Schematic of thin-walled model of arterial structure. This model is applicable when h/R << 0.1.

2. Static Pressure, Thick-Walled Cylinder Approach

The ratio of the wall thickness to the internal radius of most arteries in human circulation is approximately 0.1 or larger (62). Hence, the thin-walled, circularly cylindrical pressure vessel assumption is generally violated when applied to blood vessels, particularly those with atherosclerosis. Bergel (57,63) developed an expression for the incremental elastic modulus, E_{inc}, of an arterial segment modeled as a thick-walled, homogeneous, isotropic tube, assuming that the vessel segment is tethered and that the only load applied to the segment is the static internal pressure (pressure on the outer adventitial surface is assumed to be zero). This relationship is expressed as (57,62):

$$E_{inc} = \frac{2(1-\mu^2)\, R_1^2 R_2\, \Delta p}{(R_2^2 - R_1^2)\, \Delta R} \qquad (4)$$

μ is the Poisson's ratio and R_1 and R_2 are the internal and external radius of the vessel, respectively, Δp is the transmural pressure gradient, and R is the radial location at any point in the arterial wall. This situation is shown in Figure 3b. Note that for a vessel of constant length (i.e., tethered) and constant wall volume (i.e., incompressible, $\mu = 0.5$) the quantity $(R_2^2 - R_1^2)$ is a constant.

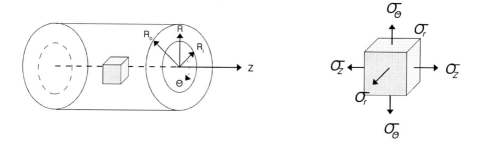

Figure 3b.   Schematic of thick-walled model of arterial structure.   This model is applicable when $h/R \geq 0.1$. This relationship assumes that the vessel material is linearly elastic, homogeneous, isotropic, and incompressible.

In applying the thick-walled formulations for the mechanical analysis of blood vessels, it is necessary to measure the transmural pressure along with the external and internal radius instantaneously. For in-vitro experiments, it is the usual practice to measure the external radius and compute the internal radius by invoking the incompressibility assumption and measuring the volume of the vessel segment. In the case of in vivo experiments, the internal radius is calculated with the assumption of uniform wall thickness and that the wall volume remains a constant. To demonstrate this approach, Bergel subjected excised canine blood vessel segments to static transmural pressures ranging up to 240 mm Hg. Bergel's results demonstrated the incremental elastic modulus increased monotonically with increases in transmural pressure. Results from other studies using canine thoracic and abdominal aortae as well as carotid and femoral arteries yielded magnitudes of E_{inc} of about 1.0×10^6 dynes/cm^2 at a transmural pressure of 40 mm Hg to about 20.0×10^6 dynes/cm^2 at a transmural pressure of 240 mm Hg.

3. *Pulse Wave Velocity Approach*

Pressure pulses generated by the heart during the contraction-relaxation cycle travel through the vessel wall as pressure waves. The velocity of the pressure pulse wave is a function of the arterial material property, the properties of blood (density and viscosity coefficient) and the wall thickness-to-lumen radius ratio. The wave velocity (c_o) of a pressure pulse traveling in a thin-walled, homogeneous, linearly elastic cylinder containing an incompressible, inviscid fluid can be expressed by the Moens-Korteweg equation (8,61):

$$C_o = \sqrt{\frac{Eh}{2\rho R}} \qquad (5)$$

where E is the elastic modulus, h is the tube thickness, ρ is the density of blood, and R is the mean radius of the tube. In many instances, C_o, h, ρ, and R can be measured or assumed, allowing estimation of elastic modulus (E) for a given segment. In-vivo measurements have shown that the pressure pulse wave velocity is on the order of 10 m/s. This approach has been successfully employed to study changes in arterial elasticity as a function of age, hypertension, diabetes, and atherosclerosis (8, 64). Once again, such an approach will yield information only about global changes in material properties in the vessel segment under investigation.

4. *Analytical Determination of Stress-Strain (Constitutive) Relationships*

The elastic behavior of the vessel walls have also been described in terms of strain energy density functions, experimentally determined via uniaxial and multiaxial force-deformation testing of vessel strips or intact vascular segments. The strain energy density function represents the strain energy input to the specimen per unit volume of the tissue to achieve a given deformation. The strain energy density function is a function of strain components, and differentiation of the strain energy density function yields the stress components (34,59). The strain energy density functions for arterial tissue derived from biaxial and triaxial tests have been represented as polynomial, exponential or logarthmic functions. These analysis have included several assumptions including: ideal cylindrical geometry, material homogeneity, cylindrically orthotropic behavior, negligible shear stress and strain , and the definition of hyperelasticity (33). However, in such formulations, a number of coefficients are required. Attributing physical meaning to these coefficients is not always possible.

5.   Parametric Techniques

In order to avoid complicated constitutive relationships, minimize geometrical measurements, and make comparisons independent of vessel, species, and age, several parameters have been proposed as a measure of vessel stiffness. Peterson, et al.(65) proposed a pressure-strain elastic modulus given by the relationship:

$$E_p = (\frac{\Delta p}{\Delta R})R_o \quad (6)$$

where E_p is the pressure modulus, Δp and ΔR are the pressure increment and corresponding change in radius, and R_o is the initial radius. Other parameters which have been used include vascular compliance $(\Delta V/V_o\Delta p)$and velocity of pulse wave propagation (see above). Hayashi (33) points out that parametric measures typically represent the structural stiffness of the vessel, and do not rigorously reflect the inherent elastic properties of the vessel wall. In addition, the magnitudes of these parameters depend upon the transmural pressure increment.

Since the pressure diameter-relationship of blood vessels is non-linear, as discussed earlier, Hayashi (33) proposed the use of a dimensionless stiffness parameter, β , defined by the relationship:

$$\ln(\frac{P}{P_s}) = \beta(\frac{D}{D_s} - 1) \quad (7)$$

where P_s is the standard pressure (typically 100 mm Hg) and D_s is the vessel diameter at the standard pressure. As will be discussed below, with the measurement of transmural pressure and the vessel diameter as a function of time, the above parameter may be used for computation of normal structural stiffness and its changes with diseased states.

6. *Dynamic Analysis*

If the blood vessel wall was composed of a pure elastic material, an instantaneous deformation is expected in response to an applied load. A measurable time, however, is required after the load is applied before the steady state deformation is attained in blood vessels. Such a response is due to the viscoelastic nature of the arterial wall material. Viscoelastic materials exhibit both creep (continuing extension due to constant load) and stress relaxation (stress decay at constant extension).

To determine the elastic modulus of viscoelastic material under static conditions, an interval of time must be allowed before the vessel will attain its steady state radius after the transmural pressure is applied. Bergel (57) determined that in most cases, no further expansion occurred approximately two minutes after the application of the transmural pressure in canine blood vessels.

The static elastic modulus by itself contains no information about the time-dependent (viscoelastic) behavior of the arterial wall, but a measure of viscoelasticity can be obtained by applying sinusoidal pressure and monitoring the resulting deformation (63). In the case of dynamic loading with a sinusoidally varying transmural pressure, even though the vessel radius will also exhibit a sinusoidal deformation, there will be a time lag between the applied pressure and the corresponding deformation. Hence under dynamic loading, the ratio of stress to strain becomes a complex number which characterizes variations in amplitude and phase lag. This ratio is known as the complex viscoelastic modulus (E_c), which is frequency-dependent. The magnitude of E_c (or $|E_c|$) represents the ratio of the amplitude of the imposed sinusoidal pressure to resulting radial deformation. The phase lag between the pressure and arterial deformation is termed ϕ, and thus E_c is properly expressed as (63):

$$E_c = |E_c|e^{j\phi}$$

(8)

where $j = \sqrt{-1}$. The real component of E_c ($|E_c| \cos \phi$) is sometimes called the dynamic elastic modulus and represents the behavior of the elastic elements of the arterial wall. The imaginary component of E_c ($j|E_c| \sin \phi$), by comparison, is used to characterize the viscous elements of the arterial wall.

In-vitro dynamic analysis, in which a sinusoidal pressure was superimposed on a mean static pressure of 100mm Hg, resulted in an increased dynamic elastic modulus at a frequency of 2 Hz compared to the corresponding static data. The dynamic elastic modulus of the muscular vessels such as the abdominal aorta, femoral and carotid arteries were about 1.2 times that of the corresponding static elastic modulus, whereas for the thoracic aorta, the ratio was found to be about 1.1(63). However, the dynamic elastic modulus was observed to be constant with further increase in frequency. In dynamic tests with a periodic (sinusoidal) loading, the delay inherent in viscous behavior prevents distension from reaching as high a peak as it does in static tests and thus the dynamic elastic modulus tends to be larger than the corresponding static values. Experiments (45,63,66) showed that the viscous component is only about 9 to 12 percent of the corresponding elastic component.

7. Finite Element Analysis

Although the preceding biomechanical analysis provide a reasonable first approximation to determining material properties in normal arteries, they are nonetheless limited by the mechanical complexity of actual arterial tissue. Moreover, the morphological variability exhibited by atherosclerotic arterial segments further confounds the reliability of conventional biomechanical analysis. Many of the shortcomings of conventional approaches of analyzing blood vessel rheology can be overcome with finite element analysis (FEA) techniques, provided that a suitable model of vascular structure is available. The FE method is a powerful numerical technique for solving physical problems such as the regional distribution of stress, or, conversely, elastic properties in a complex structure.

In FEA, the morphological details of the irregular geometry of vessel segments, if available, can be incorporated into a structural model of the study vessel. The complex three-dimensional (3D) geometry of vascular structure is subdivided to a configuration of component "finite elements" to reduce the mathematical complexity of the problem. The spatial coordinates of the corners of the finite elements (or "nodes") define the geometry of the vessel segment. The transmural pressure and appropriate boundary conditions are specified as a part of the FE analysis. A stress-strain relationship, governing mechanical behavior, is assigned to each element, and then mechanical principles are applied to each element, resulting in a set of simultaneous equations. Because the solutions obtained for any given subunit must be compatible with the solutions obtained for the neighboring elements, an iterative solution scheme is typically used. The equations are solved with a high speed digital computer. The accuracy of the FEA solution is directly related to the number of elements comprising the model and the complexity of the material laws (constitutive equations) assigned to each element .

Using this approach, regional variations in the material properties or spatial distribution of wall stress can be estimated. The FE technique has also been employed in analyzing the local changes in material properties and stresses with simulated atherosclerotic plaques (67). The predicted displacements of the nodes in response to a specified increment of pressure may readily be determined. Similarly time-dependent mechanical behavior (i.e., viscoelasticity) may be studied with the technique. Extensive applications of the finite element technique to analyze the vessel mechanics are summarized in (7). The application of the finite element method for vessel mechanics has included the incorporation of finite strain, hyperelastic behavior, and, more recently, to include tissue fluid motion by employing poroplastic constitutive laws.

III. ARTERIAL WALL PROPERTIES IN AGING AND DISEASE
A. Effects of Aging

Studies investigating the effects of aging on human vessels without cardiovascular disease indicate a loss of compliance and a corresponding increase in the inherent stiffness of the arterial structures. Kalath, et al., (68) assessed the pressure-strain modulus, as well as the circumferential elastic modulus based on thin-walled pressure vessel theory in humans as a function of age. Their results demonstrated that arteries became stiffer with age, and attributed the stiffening with increased deposition of circumferentially oriented collagen in the media with age. Buntin and Silver (60), using the same technique, reported that the stiffness of common carotid and femoral arteries increased rapidly with age as compared to the popliteal and tibial arteries. Kawasaki , et al., (69) report similar stiffening of the arteries with age, however, such stiffening was found to be significant in the deeper elastic arteries, with considerable variation reported for peripheral muscular arteries. Increased stiffness and decreased compliance of vascular segments have also been reported by Langewouters et al. (70-73), amongst others. These studies suggest that changes in the material properties of human arteries depend on the location of the arteries under study (e.g., peripheral arteries tend to be stiffer than the primary elastic arteries) and due to changes in the composition of the arteries as a function of age. In assessing the changes in vessel material properties with age, it is important to differentiate changes attributable to age from those changes more properly associated with human development and growth. Since humans cease to grow after sexual maturity, material properties of vascular segments in the aged must be compared with those of fully grown adults (74). Furthermore, it is also important to differentiate the effects of atherosclerosis and hypertension from changes in material properties due to age alone.

B.   Effects of Atherosclerosis

A number of attempts have been made to analyze the mechanical behavior of the arterial wall at various stages of atherosclerotic plaque development. These studies have included the assessment of both inherent material stiffness (e.g., E_{inc}) and structural stiffness parameters (e.g., β). Tests have included mechanical testing of specimen strips, measurement of pressure-diameter relationships in-vitro, pulse wave velocity measurements and ultrasonic measurements in-vivo. Reported results, however, have been conflicting and inconclusive (33). In general, these studies demonstrate that the wall thickness and structural stiffness increase with atherosclerosis (33,64,73,75). Farrar, et al. (64) attribute the increase in structural stiffness primarily to a concomitant increase in wall thickness. With respect to elastic modulus, several studies report an increase with atherosclerosis (13,76,77), whereas others reported a decrease in elastic modulus (12,64,78) with atherosclerosis. A number of different reasons for such conflicting results have been forwarded including: variations in measurement techniques, methods of analysis, vessel and species differences.

The material stiffness will also depend upon the composition and the stage of development of the atheromatous plaque. Composition (i.e, whether it is cellular, hypocellular or calcified) as well as morphology (i.e, eccentric, concentric, or complicated) play a significant role in determining mechanical properties of vessel segments. As atherogenesis is a diffuse and highly variable process in which lesion composition and distribution vary as a function of both axial and circumferential location within a segment (26,54) , the utility of site-specific measurements in atherosclerotic segments is debatable.

Direct measurement and FE analysis techniques have been employed to delineate the causes for mechanical rupture of atherosclerotic plaques (15,16,18,30,31) Other mechanical tests reported on atheroma include those of Castle and Grow (10). Lee, et al. (30) performed dynamic mechanical testing on isolated fibrous caps classified on the basis histological composition. It was determined that hypocellular caps were 1-2 times stiffer than cellular caps, and calcified caps were 4-5 times stiffer. Fibrous plaque caps also demonstrated an increase in stiffness with increased frequency of loading ranging from 0.5 to 10 Hz. Cheng, et al. (15) employed FE analysis to calculate the circumferential stress distribution in histological specimens of spontaneously ruptured coronary atherosclerotic lesions and compared the corresponding stress magnitudes to stable control lesions. Their analysis suggested that circumferential tensile stress concentrations in atherosclerotic plaques may play an important role in plaque rupture and subsequent myocardial infarction. Loree et al. (18) also employed the FE analysis as well as static mechanical testing in order to understand the mechanics of plaque rupture due to physiological loading. Such analysis may also be potentially useful in understanding the behavior of plaques subjected to complex mural stresses generated during balloon angioplasty (22).

C.   Effects of Hypertension

Chronic elevated blood pressure (hypertension) appears to elicit a smooth muscle response resulting in alterations in wall thickness, as well as passive mechanical properties of the arterial wall. Several studies in the large arteries of hypertensive subjects have shown an increase in the elastic modulus of arterial tissue (11, 79). Imura et al., (75) also showed that the pressure-strain modulus (E_p) of the human abdominal aorta is significantly larger in hypertensive subjects. Vaishnav et al. (32), on the other hand, reported that the ratio of stress and extension ratio was approximately the same in hypertensive and normotensive animals in the circumferential direction. More recently, Matsumoto and Hayashi (80) demonstrated that experimentally induced hypertension in the rat thoracic aorta resulted in: rapid wall thickness increase; wall stress was maintained at a normal level; and the incremental elastic modulus gradually equilibrated to that of the normal level. It has been demonstrated that aging, atherosclerosis, and hypertension alter the mechanical properties of the vasculature and that these alterations are quite complex in nature. Demonstrated alterations are a function of species, vascular bed, prevailing blood chemistry, as well as the time course of development. 3D reconstruction of arterial segments in-vivo obtained with sophisticated imaging modalities together with FE analysis may be a viable means in delineating the effects of each of the factors contributing to alteration of vascular mechanical properties. Due to the confounding effects of these processes, however, carefully designed experiments will need to be conducted to identify the unique contribution of the individual factors to altering vascular material properties.

IV.   HIGH RESOLUTION ULTRASOUND AND POTENTIAL APPLICATIONS TO VASCULAR MECHANICS

A.   Transcutaneous Ultrasound

Ultrasound imaging technologies have enjoyed an increasingly prominent role in the study of vascular mechanics. Transcutaneous vascular ultrasound modalities have the distinct advantage of allowing non-invasive, real-time assessment of vascular geometry. This attribute has facilitated study of vascular mechanical behavior in clinical and in-vivo animal experimental models. Farrar et al. (8) used ultrasound techniques to evaluate early atherosclerotic changes in the elastic properties of the carotid arteries of atherosclerotic monkeys. Megerman et al. (58) used a non-invasive ultrasonic "echo-tracking" system to study non-linear arterial compliance in dogs. Kalath et al. (68) describe the application of ultrasound imaging techniques to the non-invasive study of elastic arterial properties. Kawasaki et al. (69) evaluated age-dependent changes in human peripheral artery stiffness Buntin and Silver (60) provide a comprehensive review of ultrasound-based assessment of peripheral arterial properties. They conclude that transcutaneous ultrasound techniques provide a versatile, accurate means of measuring and quantifying vascular morphology.

Although transcutaneous ultrasound has great practical utility and does not disturb the vessel under study, this approach suffers a number of drawbacks. Image resolution is somewhat limited by the relatively low frequency of these devices (3.5 - 7.5 MHZ). Consequently, two-point structural resolution is often on the threshold of detection for some physiologically important deformations. Likewise, physical constraints of ultrasound energy, such as penetration depth, refraction, scattering, shadowing, and angle of incidence, can limit ability of ultrasound to accurately visualize pertinent vascular morphology. These shortcomings are less of a concern in superficial vessels, which can be imaged in the near field of the transducer.

B. Intravascular Ultrasound Imaging (IVUS)

Intravascular ultrasound (IVUS) is an emerging, catheter-based imaging modality that provides real-time, high resolution [typical two-point structural resolution is approximately 0.1 mm (axial) by 0.25 mm (lateral):] images of vascular structure in transverse cross-section (Figure 4).

IVUS devices owe their high resolution images to high-frequency (20-40 MHZ) piezoelectric transducers, which are incorporated into the distal catheter tip in either a phased-array or rotating element configuration. Transducer orientation is such that IVUS provides two-dimensional (2D) imaging in a plane perpendicular to the longitudinal axis of the catheter. Newer "forward-looking" IVUS designs are currently under development (82). The outer diameter of current IVUS catheters ranges from 1.0 mm to 2.7 mm, allowing insertion and utilization in variety of arterial beds. Due to the low profile of the

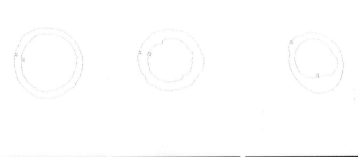

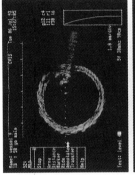

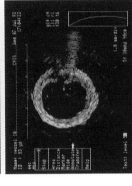

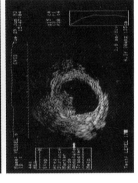

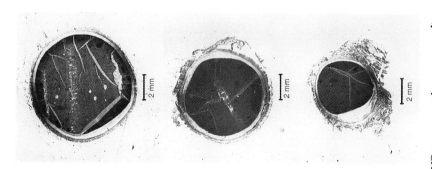

Figure (4a). 2D IVUS images with corresponding manually traced contours and (4b): histological sections (first, second, and third columns, respectively). Image and histological data depicts a normal arterial cross-section (row 1) diffusely fibro-atherosclerotic cross-section (row 2), and a complicated atherosclerotic lesion (row 3).

catheter tip, properly sized IVUS devices do not appreciably alter arterial wall mechanics in-situ.   IVUS images provide several advantages over the angiographic imaging of vascular beds: angiography requires x-ray exposure and associated risks; the radiopaque dye infusion may also alter the cardiac function and hence the coronary arteries; it has also been demonstrated that the plaque deposition is more diffuse than what is observed in angiograms.

IVUS imaging provides information on vascular segment morphology, tissue composition of the plaque and pathophysiological data after interventions. Rudimentary determination of vascular tissue composition and/or mechanical properties can be directly obtained from IVUS image data. Gussenhoven et al. (83,84) report a correlation between characteristics of high resolution IVUS images and corresponding histology of normal vascular segments. They were able to distinguish between elastin and muscular tissue based upon qualitative image interpretation. Similarly, IVUS images of atherosclerotic lesions were highly correlated with corresponding histology. In-vitro IVUS images of vascular specimens were also compared with histological analysis by Nishimura et al. (85). A high correlation between the morphology and composition depicted in the IVUS images and histological slides was found. They also observed that atherosclerotic plaques were readily visualized, but could not always be differentiated from the underlying media. Lee et al. (55) employed IVUS images on autopsy specimens with atheroma caps and classified the same as nonfibrous, fibrous and calcified based on ultrasound image appearance. Mechanical testing of the same specimens showed an increase in the elastic modulus of these classes and these results suggested that important biomechanical behavior can be predicted directly from IVUS imaging.

Intravascular   ultrasound   imaging provides significant advantages over conventional angiography. IVUS following angioplasty often reveals extensive atheroma bulk not depicted angiographically. A number of workers have suggested IVUS to be more sensitive than angiography for detecting the presence and extent of atheroma (86-88). Similar conclusions of a more complete quantitative and qualitative description of plaque geometry and composition after balloon angioplasty were also arrived at by Honye et al. (89). These studies also demonstrated the utility of IVUS for visualizing angioplasty-induced arterial trauma.

IVUS images are also being utilized in the tissue characterization of atherosclerotic plaques in order to differentiate the various components in the plaque and distinguish between normal and diseased arteries(90). This approach typically involves quantitation of the energy content of the backscattered ultrasound beam along a defined trajectory. Ng et al. (91) characterized coherent backscattered energy to differentiate plaque types of differing composition. IVUS imaging modality with tissue characterization and mechanical analysis has potential to improve our understanding of plaque development and efficacy of pharmacological and mechanical interventions.

C.   3D Reconstruction of Vascular Ultrasound Images

Since ultrasound images are confined to a single 2D scanning sector, the longitudinal extent and distribution of lesion/wall morphology is ambiguous. These shortcomings have been resolved, to a certain extent, via development of three-dimensional (3D) imaging techniques, which integrate a sequence of discrete two-dimensional images into a comprehensive rendering of vascular structure. Image data along with information regarding the spatial location from which a given image plane was collected may be assimilated via computer-intensive image processing algorithms to provide 3D renderings in wireframe, surface mapped, or volumetric formats. Three-dimensional reconstructions of vascular morphology, in turn, can be used to analyze mechanical behavior.

3D reconstruction strategies have been developed for both transcutaneous and IVUS imaging modalities. Transcutaneous 3D ultrasound imaging of vascular structure requires knowledge of the spatial location and orientation of the hand held transducer. This has been accomplished via containing probe motion to a single degree of freedom (generally parallel to the longitudinal axis of the test segment (92) , the use of mechanical registration systems (93,94), or incorporation of sophisticated position registration sensors into the hand held probe (95-97) . Although more sophisticated methods have been developed, spatial orientation of IVUS images typically involves motorized catheter withdrawal at a constant speed (i.e., the so- called "timed pullback" technique). By withdrawing the IVUS catheter along the longitudinal axis of the vessel at a constant rate, a sequence of spatially related, tomographic IVUS images may be obtained. Knowing the spatial relationship of each image plane to its neighbors, allows the serial tomographic sections to be assembled in a manner providing a volumetric representation of the entire vascular segment. Such IVUS three-dimensional reconstructions (3DR) have been shown to completely characterize the morphology and composition of the arterial segment (Figure 5) (98-102) .

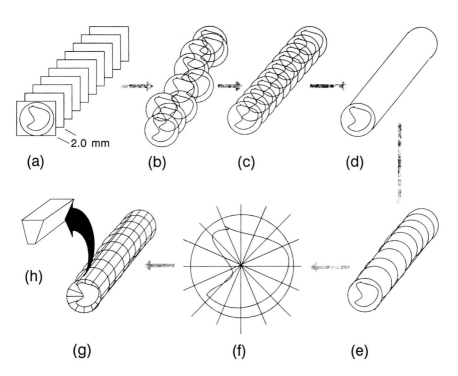

Figure 5. Flow chart for timed-pullback 3DR of IVUS data. (See text for details)

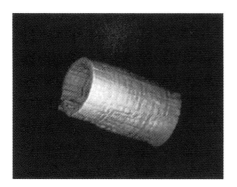 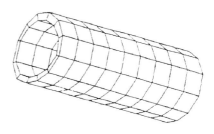

Figure 6. A typical 3D reconstruction of a segment of an in-vitro human peripheral arterial segment obtained from IVUS images employing a constant pullback technique. On the left is a voxel rendering of this structure, and on the right is the partition finite element FE model.

Discretization of the IVUS 3DR into finite elements, in turn, provides the basis for geometrically accurate models of arterial structure required by FEA techniques (Figure 6). A number of studies have been reported on computer-aided 3D reconstruction of the morphology of vascular segments from IVUS images (82,91,98,100,102). Employing a constant pullback technique and with the aid of a digital computer, a series of two-dimensional IVUS images are assembled to create a three-dimensional depiction of the vascular segment. Both sagittal and cylindrical display formats have been utilized, facilitating analysis of dissections and plaque fractures with the former and enhanced analysis of endovascular prostheses with the latter format (100). Kitney et al. (103) present a voxel based computer algorithm for 3D reconstruction and display of vascular segments from catheter-mounted ultrasound probes. Roelandt et al. (102) point out some of the specific limitations in the 3D reconstruction techniques from IVUS images because the true spatial position of the imaging catheter tip is not recorded and the complexity of curvature the vessels. Wiet et al. (104) demonstrated that the volumetric error of IVUS 3D renderings increases as vessel radius of curvature decreases (Figure 7)

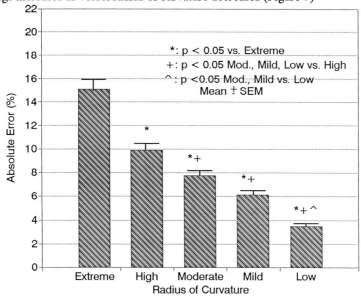

Figure 7. Effect of vessel curvature on volumetric accuracy of 3DR.

D. Finite Element Analysis of 3D Vascular Structures

The mechanical properties of atherosclerotic arterial segments vary depending upon the regional distribution of atheroma composition and morphology. A drawback of the present measurement techniques used to assess the pressure-diameter relationship of atherosclerotic vessels is that geometrical measurements obtained at localized sites in the segment may not reflect the regional variations in the vessel elasticity. Characterization of segmental morphology via high-resolution ultrasound imaging and subsequent 3D reconstruction offers specific advantages over conventional single-site measurement techniques. Using this approach, morphologically accurate 3D reconstructions can be reproducibly obtained in-vivo with a relatively minimal invasive procedure. Given geometrically accurate 3D models of vascular structure formulated at specific times in the cardiac cycle along with the measured transmural pressure at these points in time, comprehensive information of 3D deformation is available for FE analysis.

Assessment of vascular material properties using the FE analysis is schematically shown in Figure 8. This technique, similar to that described by McPherson et al. (94), begins with the assumption of a constitutive relationship for the vascular wall. With assumed material properties, the FE analysis is performed on the early geometry (3D geometry at time step 1) and the computer predicted deformation is compared with the actual deformation in time step 2. Employing an optimization algorithm, the assumed material property is adjusted such that the computer predicted deformation agrees with the actual deformation with minimal error. By optimizing for material properties on an elemental basis, regional variation in the material properties can be assessed and may be potentially applied for analysis of plaque morphology and vascular reactivity.

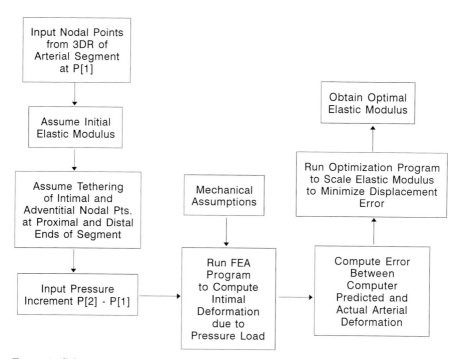

Figure 8. Schematic of a finite element analysis and optimization algorithm to estimate the material constants for a vascular segment.

As a preliminary demonstration of the potential of this technique, we performed such an analysis on human peripheral arterial specimens with varying degrees of atherosclerosis obtained at autopsy (105). The specimens, approximately 2 cm long were mounted in a specially designed chamber with both ends fixed to simulate vascular tethering. In this study, IVUS images were obtained using a timed pullback technique at transmural pressures ranging from 80 to 160 mm Hg at equal increments. Subsequently the specimens were prepared for histological examination and regionally classified as predominantly normal or atherosclerotic. An independent FE analysis was performed on the 3D models (partitioned into 120 finite elements) to assess for the material properties of the specimens as described above. In the analysis, we distinguished between normal pressure loads (80 to 120 mm Hg) and hypertensive loads (120 to 160 mm Hg). We assumed an isotropic, homogeneous, and step-wise linear material properties for the vessel in this analysis. Our results showed that the elastic modulus for the non-diseased region were inherently stiffer than those of the atherosclerotic regions for both normal and hypertensive pressure loads. These results agreed with previously published results as discussed by Hayashi (33). The elastic moduli both in the non-diseased and atherosclerotic regions were higher at the hypertensive pressure loads compared to the lower pressures indicating the stiffening of the vessels at higher transmural pressures. The results from this analysis on autopsy specimens are summarized in Figure 9.

We have also demonstrated the potential application of this technique using in-vivo IVUS imaging and simultaneous hemodynamic measurements. Here, we obtained sequential IVUS images using the timed pullback technique from the descending aorta of dogs which were used to create 3D reconstructions of segmental morphology. Using simultaneous transmural pressure measurements, we performed the FE analysis described above with anisotropic constitutive relationship (106). Our results were in close agreement with those reported by (47).

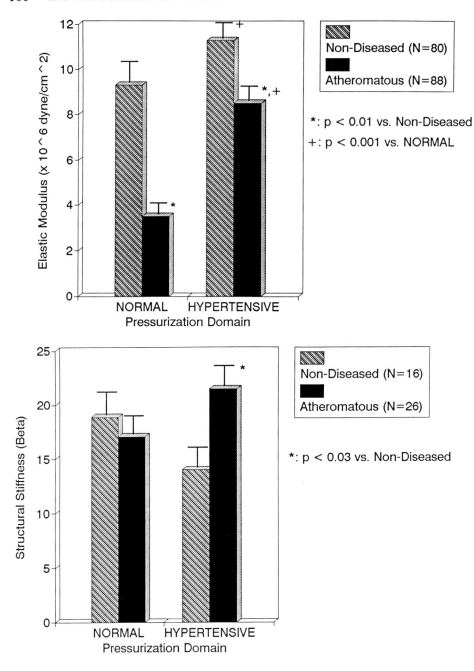

Figure 9. Results of in-vitro mechanical property assessment of autopsy specimens of human peripheral arteries using IVUS images and finite element analysis described in the text (a) Estimated elastic modulus vs. pressurization domain as a function of disease state. (b) Structural stiffness (β) vs. pressurization domain as a function of disease state.

(b)

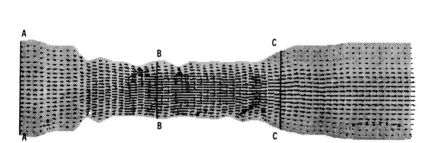

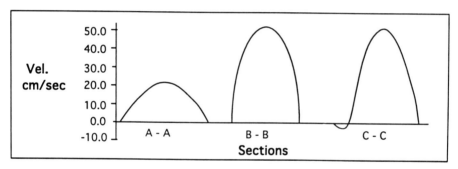

Figure 10. Analysis of flow dynamics within a vascular segment with an artificially induced stenosis with a lumen area reduction of forty percent. The velocity profiles at the throat and distal to the stenosis computed from the flow dynamic analysis are also represented in the figure.

Given the morphologically realistic 3D reconstruction of the luminal surface along with pressure and point velocity measurements, these data can also be used to analyze the flow dynamics within the segment in detail as a function of plaque morphology (107). The details of the wall shear stress distribution in the vicinity of the plaques can be analyzed using computational fluid dynamic analysis (CFD) in order to delineate the effect of flow dynamics on the atheroma formation. A typical example of an artificially induced stenosis reconstructed from IVUS images is shown in Figure 10. The artery was constricted with an elastic band placed around the exposed artery to induce an approximately forty percent area reduction in the segment. Simultaneous pressure and point velocity measurements using a Doppler probe were obtained proximal and distal to the segment along with the IVUS images for the 3D reconstruction. A commercially available computational fluid dynamics package, FLOW 3D was employed to analyze the velocity profiles and wall shear stresses in the vicinity of the stenosis with the measured pressure and velocity data being applied as boundary conditions. The computed velocity profiles at the throat and distal to the stenosis s are also shown in Figure 10. Computations of the wall shear stress as well as regions of flow stasis and separation from such an analysis can potentially used in long-term studies in order to correlate the effect of hemodynamics on the plaque formation and development.

V. SUMMARY

Analysis of vascular wall rheology in normal and pathological conditions may play a vital role in early diagnosis and treatment of vascular disease. The following conclusions can be drawn from the preceding review of vascular mechanics presented in this chapter:

1.   Vascular wall material is an inhomogeneous composite of elastin, collagen and smooth muscle exhibiting a non-linear, cylindrically orthotropic stress-strain relationship. However, within the range of physiologic deformation, assumption of step-wise linear, homogeneous, isotropic elastic property for the vessel wall may be reasonable in our ability to differentiate between normal and pathological segments.

2.   In-vitro and in-vivo mechanical analysis have established changes in vascular reactivity with age, hypertension, and atherosclerosis. Most of the experimental site-specific measurements employed in the mechanical analysis do not yield   information on regional variation in material properties with diffuse atherosclerotic disease.

3.   High resolution ultrasound imaging techniques, along with hemodynamic measurements, may be exploited in the regional analysis of vascular reactivity with the onset of atherosclerosis. Computer-aided 3D reconstruction of these images can provide morphologically accurate 3D models of the vascular segments at different times in the cardiac cycle. As has been demonstrated with some preliminary studies in this area, the combination of high resolution ultrasound images and hemodynamic measurements can be potentially used for mechanical analysis of vascular reactivity.

4.   These analysis methods may also be employed in selecting and determining the efficacy of pharmacological and mechanical interventions on arresting and/or reversing atheromatous plaque progression.

In summary, an understanding of the mechanical behavior of vascular tissue in the presence of cardiovascular disease requires analysis of the complex interaction between the vessel wall and blood flow. With the advent of sophisticated imaging modalities, it is now possible to obtain morphologically realistic 3D geometries of vascular segments throughout the cardiac cycle.

These analysis techniques also provide information on the regional variation and distribution of vascular reactivity due to diffuse disease processes. A detailed description of the distribution of fluid mechanical and intramural stresses may be important to studying the cellular response to these stimuli. Such analysis hold promise for detecting the onset of diseased states in their early stages so that appropriate pharmacological, behavioral, or mechanical interventions can be initiated to modulate the effects of the disease process. Application of advanced imaging engineering analysis tools to cardiovascular medical problems is a promising avenue of research that is likely to find role in the future of clinical patient care.

Acknowledgment:

Partial support of this work by the Chicago Heart Association, the Feinberg Cardiovascular Research Institute, and the National Institutes of Health (NHLBI HL 46550) is gratefully acknowledged.

References

1. Bergel DH. The properties of blood vessels. In: Fung YC, Perrone N, Anliker M (eds), Biomechanics: Its foundations and objectives. Prentice-Hall, 1972; 105-140.
2. Patel DJ, Vaishnav RN. The rheology of large blood vessels. In: Bergel DH (ed)Cardiovascular fluid dynamics. Academic Press, New York, 1972; pp 2-65.
3. Canfield TR, Dobrin PB. Static elastic properties of blood vessels. In: Skalak R, Chien S (eds)Handbook of bioengineering. McGraw-Hill, 1987; pp 16.1-16.27.
4. Fry DL. Acute vascular endothelial changes associated with increased blood velocity gradients. Circulation Research 1968; 22: 165-197.
5. Fry DL, Vaishnav RN. Mass transport in the arterial wall. In: Fry DL, Vaishnav RN (eds),Basic hemodynamics and its role in disease processes. University Park Press 1980; pp 425-482.
6. Nerem RM, Levesque MJ. Fluid mechanics in atherosclerosis. In: Chien S, Skalak R (eds)Handbook of bioengineering. McGraw-Hill, 1987
7. Simon, BR, Kaufman, MV, McAfee, MA, Baldwin AL. Finite element models for arterial wall mechanics. ASME J. Biomechanical Engineering 1987; 115: 489-496.
8. Farrar DJ, Green HD, Bond MG, Wagner, WD, Gobbe RA. Aortic pulse wave velocity, elasticity, and composition in a nonhuman primate model of atherosclerosis. Circulation Research 1978; 43: 52-62.
9. Middleman S. The cardiovascular system. In: Transport phenomena in the cardiovascular system. Wiley-Interscience 1972; pp 1-49.
10. Castle WD, Gow BS. Changes in the microindentation properties of aortic intimal surface during cholesterol feeding of rabbits. Atherosclerosis 1983; 47: 251-261.
11. Cox RH, Bagshaw RJ. Effects of hypertension and its reversal on canine arterial wall properties. Hypertension 1988; 12: 301-309.
12. Haut RC, Garg BD, Metke M, Josa, M., Kaye, MP Mechanical properties of the canine aorta following hypercholesterolemia. ASME J. Biomechanical Engineering 1980; 102: 98-102
13. Hayashi K., Takamizawa K, Nakamura T, Kato T, Tsushima N. Effects of elastase on the stiffness and elastic properties of arterial walls in cholesterol-fed rabbits. Atherosclerosis 1987; 66: 259-267.
14. Liu ZR, Ting CT, Zhu S, Yin FC. Aortic compliance in human hypertension. Hypertension 1989; 14: 129-136.
15. Cheng GC, Loree HM, Kamm RD, Fishbein FC, Lee RT. Distribution of circumferential stress in ruptured and stable atherosclerotic lesions: A structural analysis with histopathologic correlation. Circulation 1993; 87: 1179-1187.
16. Loree HM, Kamm RD, Stringfellow RG, Lee R. Effects of fibrous cap thickness on peak circumferential stress in model atherosclerotic vessels. Circulation Research 1992; 71: 850-858.
17. Loree HM, Grodzinsky AJ, Park SY, Gibson LJ, Lee RT. Static circumferential tangential modulus of human atherosclerotic tissue. J. Biomechanics, New York University Press 1994a; 27: 195-204.
18. Loree HM, Tobias BJ, Gibson LJ, Kamm RD, Small DM, Lee RT. Mechanical properties of model atherosclerotic lesion lipid pools. Arteriosclerosis & Thrombosis 1994b; 14: 230-234.
19. Richardson PD, Davies MJ, Born GV. Influence of plaque configuration and stress distribution on fissuring of coronary atherosclerotic plaques [see comments]. Lancet 2: 941-944.
20. Thubrikar MJ, Baker JW, Nolan SP. Inhibition of atherosclerosis associated with reduction of arterial intramural stress in rabbits. Arteriosclerosis 1988; 8: 410-420.
21. Lee RT, Loree HM, Cheng GC, Lieberman EH, Jaramillo N, Schoen FJ. Computational structural analysis based on intravascular ultrasound imaging before in vitro angioplasty: prediction of plaque fracture locations. Journal of the American College of Cardiology 1993; 21: 777-782.
22. Oh S, Kleinberger M, McElhaney JHA. Finite element analysis of balloon angioplasty. ASME/BED Advances in Bioengineering 1992; 22: 269-272.
23. Oktay HS, Resar J, Humphrey JD. Mechanics of conventional and thermal balloon angioplasty. ASME/BED Advances in Bioengineering 1992; 24: 305-306.
24. Glagov S, Weisenberg E, Zarins C K, Stankunavisius R, Kolettis G. Compensatory enlargement of human atherosclerotic coronary arteries. N Eng. J. Med.1987; 316: 1371-1375.
25. McPherson DD, Hiratzka LF, Lamberth WC, Brandt B, Hunt M, Kieso RA, Marcus ML, Kerber RE. Delineation of the extent of coronary atherosclerosis by high-frequency epicardial echocardiography. New England Journal of Medicine 1987a; 316:304-309.
26. Ross R. The pathogenesis of atherosclerosis. Chapter 36 in Heart Disease: A Textbook of Cardiovascular Medicine. Vol. 2., E. Braunwald, Ed., W. B. Saunders 1992; pp. 1106-1124.

27. Glagov S, Zarins C, Giddens DP, Ku DN. Hemodynamics and atherosclerosis. Insights and perspectives gained from studies of human arteries. [Review]. Archives of Pathology & Laboratory Medicine 1988; 112: 1018-1031.

28. Davies MJ, Thomas AC. Plaque fissuring- the cause of acute myocardial infarction, sudden ischemic death, and crescendo angina.[Review]. British Heart Journal 1985; 53: 363-373.

29. Briggs AD, Burleigh MC, Lendon CL, Born GVR, Davies MJ. Biochemical analysis of individual atherosclerotic plaque caps to investigate susceptibility to rupture. Biochemical Society Transactions 1988; 16:1033-1034.

30. Lee RT, Grodzinsky AJ, Frank EH, Kamm RD, Schoen FJ. Structure-dependent dynamic mechanical behavior of fibrous caps from human atherosclerotic plaques. Circulation 1991; 83: 1764-1770.

31. Lendon CL, Davies M J, Richardson P D, Born GVR. Testing of small connective tissue specimens for the determination of mechanical behavior of atherosclerotic plaques. J. Biomedical Engineering, 1993; 15: 27-33.

32. Vaishnav RN, Vassoughi J, Patel DJ, Cothran LN, Coleman BR , Ison-Franklin EL. Effect of hypertension on elasticity and geometry of aortic tissue from dogs. ASME J. Biomechanical Engineering 1990; 112: 70-74.

33. Hayashi K. Experimental approaches on measuring the mechanical properties and constitutive laws of arterial walls. ASME J. Biomechanical Engineering 1993; 115: 481-488.

34. Fung YC. Biomechanics. Mechanical Properties of Living Tissues. Springer-Verlag 1981.

35. Dewey CF, Bussolari SR, Gimbrone MA, Davies PF The dynamic response of vascular endothelial cells to fluid shear stress. Journal of Biomechanical Engineering 1981; 103: 177-185.

36. Levesque MJ, Nerem RM . The elongation and orientation of cultured endothelial cells in response to shear stress. Journal of Biomechanical Engineering 1985; 107: 341-347.

37. Burton AC. Physiology and Biophysics of the Circulation, Year Book Medical Publishers 1965.

38. Pasterkamp G, Wensing PJW, Post M J, Hillen B, Mali WPTM, Borst C. Paradoxical arterial wall shrinkage may contribute to luminal narrowing of human atherosclerotic femoral arteries. Circulation 1995; 91: 1444-1449.

39. Armentano R., Simon A, Levenson J, Chau N P, Megnien JL , Pichel, R. Mechanical pressure versus intrinsic effects of hypertension on large arteries in humans. Hypertension, 1991; 18: 657-664.

40. Carew TE, Vaishnav RN and Patel DJ. Compressibility of the arterial wall. Circulation Research 1968; 23: 61-68.

41. Chuong CJ, Fung YC. Compressibility and constitutive equation of arterial wall in radial compression experiments. J. Biomechanics 1984; 17: 35-40.

42. Weizsacker HW, Pinto, JG. Isotropy and anisotropy of the arterial wall. J Biomechanics 1988; 21: 477-487.

43. Dobrin PB. Biaxial anisotropy of dog carotid artery: Estimation of circumferential elastic modulus. J. Biomechanics 1986; 19: 351-358.

44. Patel DJ, Janicki JS. Carew TE Static anisotropic elastic properties of the aorta in living dogs. Circulation Research, 1969; 25: 765-779.

45. Patel DJ, Janicki JS, Vaishnav RN, Young, JT. Dynamic anisotropicvisco elastic properties of the aorta in living dogs. Circulation Research, 1973; 32: 93-107 .

46. Gentile BJ, Chuong CJC, Ordway GA . Regional volume distensibility of canine thoracic aorta during moderate treadmill exercise. Circulation Research 1988; 63: 1012-1019.

47. Papageorgiou GL , Jones NB. Circumferential and longitudinal viscoelasticity of human iliac arterial segments in-vitro. J. Biomedical Engineering 1988; 10: 82-90.

48. Sato M, Hayashi K, Niimi H, Moritake K, Okumura AS, Handa H . Axial mechanical properties of arterial walls and their anisotropy. Medical and Biological Engineering and Computing 1979; 17: 170-176.

49. Vassoughi J, Weizsacker HW. Elastic properties of blood vessels in simple elongation. Biomechanics: Current Interdisciplinary Research, S. M. Perren and E. Schneider, Eds., Martinus Nijhoff Publishers, Dordrecht,.1985; pp. 251-256.

50. Tanaka TT, Fung YC . Elastic and inelastic properties of the canine aorta and their variations along the aortic tree. J. Biomechanics 1974; 7: 357-370.

51. Cox, RH. Compressibilities and constitutive equation of arterial wall in radial compression experiments. J Biomechanics 1983; 17:35-40.

52. Mohan D, Melvin JW. Failure properties of passive human aortic tissue. I--uniaxial tension tests. Journal of Biomechanics 1982; 15:887-902.

53.   Mohan D, Melvin JW.   Failure properties of passive human aortic tissue. II--Biaxial tension tests. Journal of Biomechanics 1983; 16:31-44.

54.   Born GVR, and Richardson PD.   Mechanical properties of human atherosclerotic lesions. Chapter 27 in Pathobiology of the human atherosclerotic plaque. S. Glagov, W. P. Newman, S. A. Schaffer (Eds.) Springer-Verlag 1990 pp. 413-423.

55.   Lee RT, Richardson G, Loree HM, Grodzinsky AJ, Gharib SA, Schoen FJ, Pandian N.   Prediction of mechanical properties of human atherosclerotic tissue by high-frequency intravascular ultrasound imaging. An in-vitro study. Arteriosclerosis and Thrombosis 1992; 12(1): 1-5.

56.   Demer LL, Yin, FCP.   Passive biaxial mechanical properties of isolated canine myocardium. J. Physiol 1983; 339: 615-630.

57.   Bergel DH.   The static elastic properties of the arterial wall. J. Physiol 1961a; 156:445-457.

58.   Megerman J, Hasson JE, Warnock DF, L'Italien GJ, Abbott WM.   Noninvasive measurements of nonlinear arterial elasticity. Am. J. Physiol. 250 (Heart Circ. Physiol. 19) 1986; H181-H188.

59.   Hayashi K.   Fundamental and applied studies of mechanical properties of cardiovascular tissues. Biorheology 1982; 19:425-436.

60.   Buntin CM, Silver FH.   Noninvasive assessment of mechanical properties of peripheral arteries. Annals of Biomedical Engineering 1990; 18: 549-566.

61.   Chandran KB. Cardiovascular Biomechanics, New York University Press, New York, 1992.

62.   Milnor W R. Hemodynamics, Williams and Wilkins 1989.

63.   Bergel DH. The dynamic elastic properties of the arterial wall. J. Physiol. 1961b; 156:458-469.

64.   Farrar DJ, Bond M G, Sawyer JK, and Green, HD. Pulse wave velocity and morphological changes associated with early atherosclerosis progression in the aortas of cynomolgus monkeys. Cardiovascular Research 1984; 18: 107-118.

65.   Peterson LH, Jensen RE, Parnell J. Mechanical properties of arteries in-vivo. Circulation, Research 1960; 8: 622-639.

66.   Gow BS, Taylor MG. Measurement of viscoelastic properties of arteries in living dogs. Circulation Research 1968; 28: 278-292.

67.   Chandran KB, Ray G. (1982) Clinical implications of pressure deformation analysis of curved elastic tubes. Medical & Biological Engineering & Computing 1994a; 20: 145-150.

68.   Kalath S, Tsipoura P, Silver FH.   Non-invasive assessment of aortic mechanical properties. Annals of Biomedical Engineering 1986; 14: 513-524.

69.   Kawasaki T, Sasayama S, Yagi S, Asakawa T, Hirai T.   Non-invasive assessment of the age related changes in stiffness of major branches of human arteries. Cardiovascular Research 1987; 21: 678-687.

70.   Hayashi K, Handa, H Nagasawa S, Okamura A, Moritake K.   Stiffness and elastic behavior of human intracranial and extracranial arteries. J. Biomechanics 1980; 13: 175-184.

71.   Langewouters G L, Wesseling KH, and Goedhard WJA. The static elastic properties of 45 human thoracic and 20 abdominal aortas in-vitro and the parameters of a newmodel. J. Biomechanics 1984; 17: 425-435.

72   Langewouters GJ, Wesseling K H, Goedhard WJA.   Age related changes in viscoelasticity of normal and arteriosclerotic human aortas. Biomechanics: Current Interdisciplinary Research, S. M. Perren and E. Schneider, Eds., Martinus Nijhoff, Dodrecht, 1985; pp. 245-250.

73.   Hirai T, Sasayama S, Kawasaki T, Yagi S. Stiffness of systemic arteries in patients with myocardial infarction - A noninvasive method to predict severity of coronary atherosclerosis. Circulation, 1989; 89: 78-86.

74.   Harris R Aging of the cardiovascular system. in Lectures on Gerontology, Vol. I. On Biology of Ageing Part B,Viidik A. Editor, Chapter 8, Academic Press, New York.

75.   Imura T, Yamamoto K, Satoh T, Mikami T, Yasuda H. Arteriosclerotic change in the human abdominal aorta in-vivo in relation to coronary heart disease and risk factors. Atherosclerosis 1988; 73: 149-155.

76.   Pynadath T, Mukherjee, DP. Dynamic mechanical properties of atherosclerotic aorta. Atherosclerosis, 1977; 26: 311-318.

77.   Hayashi K, Ide K, Matsumoto T. Aortic walls in atherosclerotic rabbits - Mechanical study. ASME J. Biomechanical Engineering 1994; 116: 284-293.

78.   Hudetz AG, Mark G, Kovach AGB, Kerenyi T, Fody L, Monos E.   Biomechanical properties of normal and fibrosclerotic human cerebral arteries. Atherosclerosis 1981; 39: 353-365.

79.   Sharma MG, Hollis TM. Rheological properties of arteries under normal and experimental hypertension conditions. J. Biomechanics 1976; 9: 293-300.

80.   Matsumoto T, Hayashi K. Mechancical and dimensional adaptation of rat aorta to hypertension. ASME J. Biomechanical Engineering 1994; 116: 278 - 283.

81. Powalowski T, Pensko B, Trawinski Z, Malek A, Staszkiewicz W, Szostek M. Ultrasonic noninvasive examination of the human cerebrovascular system using the vascular impedance method. Pol Tyg Lek. 1989 ; 44(5):120-3

82. Evans JL, Ng K H, Vonesh M J, Kramer BL, Mills TA, Kane BJ, Aldrich WN, Jang YT, Yock PG, Rold MD, Roth SI, McPherson DD. Arterial imaging utilizing a new forward viewing intravascular ultrasound catheter. Initial studies. Circulation 1994; 89: 712-717.

83. Gussenhoven EJ, Essed CE, Lancee CT, Mastik F, Frietman P, van Egmond FC, Reiber J, Bosch H, van Urk H, Roelandt J. Arterial wall characteristics determined by intravascular ultrasound imaging: An in-vitro study. J. Am. Coll. Cardiol 1989b; 14: 947-952.

84. Gussenhoven EJ, Essed CE, Frietman P, Mastik F, Lancee C, Slager C, Serruy P, Gerritsen P, Pieterman H, Bom N. Intravascular echocardiographic assessment of vessel wall characteristics: A correlation with histology. Int J of Card Imaging, 1989a; 4(2-4):105-116

85. Nishimura RA, Edwards WD, Warnes CA, Reeder GS, Holmer DR Jr, Tajik AJ, Yock PG. Intravascular ultrasound imaging: In Vitro validation and pathologic correlation. J Am Coll Cardiol 1990:16(1):145-154.

86. Tobis JM, Mallery J, Mahon D, Gesser J, Griffith J, Bessen M, Moriuchi M, McLeay L, McRae M, Henry WL. Intravascular ultrasound imaging of human coronary arteries in-vivo. Analysis of tissue characterizations with comparison to in vitro histological specimens. Circulation 1991; I 83: 913-926.

87. Liebson PR, Klein LW. Intravascular ultrasound in coronary atherosclerosis: a new approach to clinical assessment. [Review]. American Heart Journal 1992; 123:1643-1660.

88. Waller BF, Pinkerton CA, Slack JD. Intravascular ultrasound: a histological study of vessels during life. The new 'gold standard' for vascular imaging [Review]. Circulation 1992; 85:2305-2310.

89. Honye J, Maho, DJ, Jain A, White C J, Ramee SR, Wallis JB, al-Zarka, A, Tobis JM. Morphological effects of coronary balloon angioplasty in-vivo assessed by intravascular ultrasound imaging. Circulation 1992; 85 1012-1025.

90. Linker DT, Yock PG, Gronningsaether A., Johansen E, Angelsen BAJ. Analysis of backscattered ultrasound from normal and diseased arterial wall. Int. J. of Cardiac Imaging 1989; 4: 177-185.

91. Ng K H, Evans JL, Vonesh MJ, Meyers SL, Mills TA, Kane BJ, Aldrich WN, Jang YT, Yock PG, Rold MD, Roth SI, McPherson DD. Three dimensional reconstruction and display of forward viewing intravascular ultrasound data. Circulation 1994; 89:718-723.

92. Vonesh, MJ, Mesh C, Ng KH, Blackburn DR, McPherson DD, Yao JST. Three-dimensional reconstruction of the carotid bifurcaton with vascular ultrasound using a new position registration device. Circulation 1991; 84:11-22.

93. Geiser EA, Ariet M., Conetta DA, Lupkiewicz SM, Christie LG, Conti, CR. Dynamic three-dimensional echocardiographic reconstruction of the intact human left ventricle: Technique and initial observations in patients. American Heart Journal 1982; 103:1056-1065.

94. McPherson DD, Skorton DJ, Kodiyalam S, Petree L, Noel MP, Kieso R, Kerber RE, Collins SM, Chandran KB. Finite element analysis of myocardial diastolic function using three-dimensional echocardiographic reconstructions: Application of a new method for study of acute ischemia in dogs. Circulation Research 1987b; 60: 674-682.

95. Moritz WE, Shreve PL. A microprocessor-based spatial locating system for use with diagnostic ultrasound. Proceedings IEEE 1976; 64:966-974.

96. Joskowicz G, Klicpera M, Pachinger O, Probst P, Mayr H, Kaindl F. Computer supported measurements of 2D echocardiographic images. IEEE Proceedings Computers in Cardiology 1981; 13-17.

97. King DL, King DL, Yi-Ci Shao M . Three-dimensional spatial registration and interactive display of position and orientation of real-time ultrasound images. Journal of Ultrasoud in Medicine 1990; 9:525-532.

98. Rosenfield K, Losordo DW, Ramaswamy K, Pastore JO, Langevin RE, Razvi S, Kosowsky BD, Isner JM. Three-dimensional reconstruction of human coronary and peripheral arteries from images recorded during two-dimensional intravascular ultrasound examination. Circulation 1991; 84: 1938-1956.

99. Tobis JM. Intravascular Ultrasound. A fantastic Voyage. Circulation 1991; 84: 2190-2192.

100. Rosenfield K, Kaufman J, Pieczek AM, Langevin RE Jr., Palefski PE, Razvi SA, Isner JM. Human coronary and peripheral arteries: On-line three-dimensional reconstruction from two-dimensional intravascular US scans. Radiology 1992; 184: 823-832.

101. Coy KM, Park JC, Fishbein MC, Laas T, Diamond GA, Adler L, Maurer G, Siegel RJ. In vitro validation of three-dimensional intravascular ultrasound for the evaluation of arterial injury after balloon angioplasty [see comments]. Journal of the American College of Cardiology, 1992; 20:692-700.

102. Roelandt JR, di Mario C, Pandian NG, Wenguang L, Keane D, Slager CJ, de Feyter PJ, Seruys PW. Three-dimensional reconstruction of intracoronary ultrasound images. Rationale, approaches, problems and directions. Circulation 1994; 90:1044-1055.

103. Kitney RI, Moura L, Straughan K . 3-D visualization of arterial structures using ultrasound and voxel modelling. Int. J.of Cardiac Imaging 1989; 4:135-143.

104. Wiet SP, Vonesh MJ, Waligora MJ, Kane BJ, McPherson DD. The Effect of Vascular Curvature on Three-Dimensional Reconstruction of Intravascular Ultrasound Images. (Submitted)

105. Vonesh MJ, Pinto JV, Cho CH, Pinto JV, Lee DS, Roth SI, Chandran KB, McPherson DD. Characterization of vascular mechanical properties with three-dimensional intravascular ultrasound and finite element analysis. J. Am. Coll. Cardiol 1994; 23:378A.

106. Vonesh MJ, Cho CH, Greenfield S, Kane BJ, Greene R, Chandran KB, McPherson DD. A novel method to determine in-vivo vascular anisotropic material properties using three dimensional reconstruction of intravascular ultrasound images and finite element analysis. J Invest Med 1995; 43:386A

107. Chandran KB, Vonesh MJ, Roy R, Kane BJ, Greene R, McPherson, DD. Vascular Flow dynamic analysis from intravascular ultrasound images. Medical Engineering and Physics 1996. (In Press)

QUANTITATIVE ULTRASONIC TISSUE CHARACTERIZATION WITH INTRAVASCULAR AND TRANSCUTANEOUS ULTRASOUND

Samuel A. Wickline, M.D., James G. Miller, Ph.D.
and Gregory M. Lanza, M.D., Ph.D.

Washington University School of Medicine and Department of Physics
St. Louis, Missouri U.S.A.

Contents

I. INTRODUCTION

Vascular disease is responsible for the majority of deaths in the United States from coronary artery and peripheral vascular disease, stroke, and arterial dissection or rupture. The ultimate biological behavior of atherosclerotic lesions depends not only on their extent of luminal narrowing but also on their biophysical composition and material properties. Ultrasonic tissue characterization methods may be useful for quantitative delineation of the biophysical composition and organization of normal and pathological vascular tissue.

Ultrasonic imaging with intravascular ultrasound is well suited for evaluation of atherosclerotic lesion morphology because it provides an image through the full thickness of the vessel wall that reflects local material properties and tissue organization. Intravascular ultrasound has been generally accepted in clinical practice as a technique that is more sensitive to subtle aspects of vessel morphology than is available from routine coronary angiography. Its major clinical use to date has involved assessment of coronary artery lesions after treatment with mechanical interventions such as balloon or laser angioplasty, or atherectomy. Much of this work has been performed with miniature ultrasonic transducer-tipped catheters that range in frequency from 20-30 MHz. Nevertheless, a prominent role for intravascular ultrasound in the diagnostic armamentarium of clinical cardiology has not yet been firmly established due to considerations of cost and questions of the relative value added to more conventional methods for diagnosing coronary artery disease. The purpose of this chapter is to provide a brief overview of the potential utility and limitations of intravascular and transvascular ultrasound for *quantitative* characterization of vascular tissue.

II. QUANTITATIVE TISSUE CHARACTERIZATION

Qualitative descriptions of vessel morphologic features based on conventional image data acquired from vessels imaged in vitro have been correlated with histology to provide modest insights into the scattering behavior of normal and pathologic coronary and peripheral vascular tissues.[1,2,3] Most of these studies have provided pathologic correlations of lesion type (fatty, fibrous, or calcified) with subjective classification of scattering amplitude ("hypo-echoic", "hyper-echoic", "shadowing"). Most clinicians can easily appreciate these general categories of scattering behavior without quantitative assessment and readily associate them with certain lesion types. Whether these qualitative descriptors of vessel type are sufficient to permit assessment of the biological activity of lesions, or their propensity for plaque rupture, thrombosis, occlusion and infarction is conjectural at this time, but remains a principal goal of researchers in the field.

Despite the widespread clinical application of intravascular ultrasound, surprisingly little quantitative analysis of arterial scattering behavior has been performed. Previous work by Picano et al in vitro demonstrated quantitative differences in the magnitude of scattering from pathologic components of vascular tissue such as fibrous, fatty, and calcified plaque.[4,5] Studies by Barzilai et al indicated that calcium content was a primary determinant of scattering amplitude from atherosclerotic lesions.[6]. Both of these groups used lower ultrasonic frequencies (<10 MHZ) that only permitted rough correlation of scattering behavior with plaque constituents. Lockwood et al reported some of the first quantitative measurements of ultrasonic indexes of lesion composition with the use of higher frequencies that are potentially clinically applicable.[7,8]

A. Physiologic Vascular Structure

Intravascular ultrasound images reflect vessel morphologic characteristics of composition and architecture. Normal muscular arteries (coronary, distal carotid) may exhibit either a 2 or 3 layered structure (depending on resolution of the catheter), which incorporates prominent specular reflections from the internal and external elastic laminae. For most imaging transducers, the intimal layer is too thin (50 microns or less) to be distinguished from the strong internal elastic lamina reflection, and typically only appears as a separate third layer when it is abnormally thickened.[9] However, with the use of imaging systems possessing sufficiently high frequency and resolution features, the normal intimal thickness can be determined.[10] The medial layer generally exhibits weak scattering due to the prevalence of smooth muscle cells interdigitated with only a modest amount of collagen matrix, whereas the adventitia displays greater scattering due to its more extensive collagen matrix. The walls of normal elastic arteries appear as a single "high scattering" layer due to the relatively uniform and prominent distribution of elastin and collagen. The structural components of the elastic artery comprise a highly organized arrangement of lammelae that comprise repeating modules of elastin, collagen, and smooth muscle cells[11] which obscure reflections from any discrete internal and external elastic layers.

The alignment of elastic matrix fibers such as elastin and collagen in elastic arteries produces an angle dependence of scattering, or ultrasonic anisotropy. DeKroon et al measured the anisotropic properties of normal elastic and muscular arteries at 27 MHZ and showed that both types manifest substantial directivity in terms of a Gaussian parameterization that quantifies the angle dependent change in integrated backscatter (dB/degree²).[12] Fibrous arterial lesions also exhibited angle dependent scattering behavior. Lockwood also found that both carotid and femoral arteries exhibited significant anisotropy with the use of a 50 MHZ broadband transducer.[7,8] Lockwood et al also measured backscatter coefficients (in units of steradian·mm⁻¹) from these vessel types with and without "soft plaque" and "thickened intima", and demonstrated relatively lower scattering from soft plaque than from thickened intima.

We have recently examined the quantitative relationship between the presence of elastin and collagen in vessels and backscatter amplitude to delineate the important physical features of vessels responsible for scattering behavior. Segments of arteries excised from selected anatomic sites in the vascular tree of normal pigs were insonified from the endothelial side perpendicular to circumferential orientation of vascular wall fibers with a 50 MHZ focused piezoelectric transducer. Integrated backscatter was calculated for rf data windowed from the subendothelial layer by computing the power spectrum of the gated signal, referencing the power backscattered from tissue to that returned from a stainless steel reflector (a near-perfect reflector), and then averaging the relative power (or, the backscatter transfer function) across the useful bandwidth of the transducer. The answer is expressed in decibels (dB) where negative numbers indicate that tissues exhibit lower scattering intensities than does the steel plate. Elastin and collagen contents were determined from stained sections (von Gieson and trichrome) of tissue with the use of computer-assisted planimetry.[14]

Figure 1 shows the dependence of integrated backscatter on anatomic location. Integrated backscatter increases progressively from muscular (coronary) to elastic (aorta) artery segments, with a range of backscatter values greater than 20 dB for normal vessels. An approximately linear dependence on the amount of both collagen and elastin was observed (see Figure 2), which may not be surprising for normal vessels because both of these proteins are integral and proportionate matrix components. The amount of smooth muscle cells present in the matrix is inversely related to the measurement of integrated backscatter, which is consistent with previous qualitative observations based on intravascular ultrasound images that medial layers of muscular arteries are poorly reflective. Thus, the highly reflective elements comprise fibrous matrix proteins.

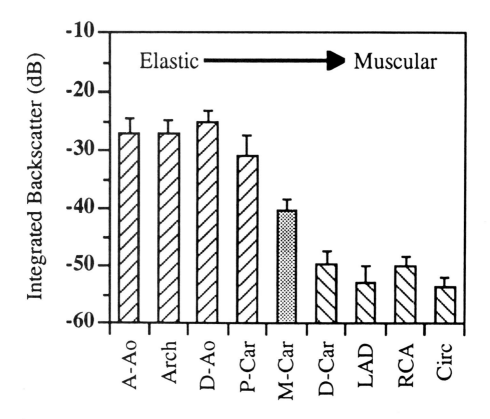

Figure 1. The dependence of backscatter from subendothelial layers of normal vascular tissue reflects anatomic location within the vascular tree. The transition from elastic to muscular arteries occurs at the mid carotid (M-Car) level. The first 3 bars are ascending (A-), Arch, and descending (D-) aorta (Ao), the next three are proximal (P-), mid (M-), and distal (D-) carotid (Car), and the final 3 are left anterior descending (LAD), right (RCA), and circumflex (Circ) coronary arteries. (With permission, from reference 13).

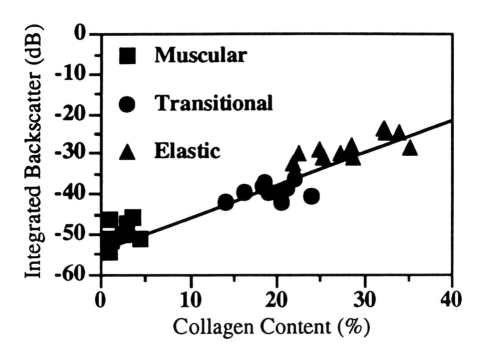

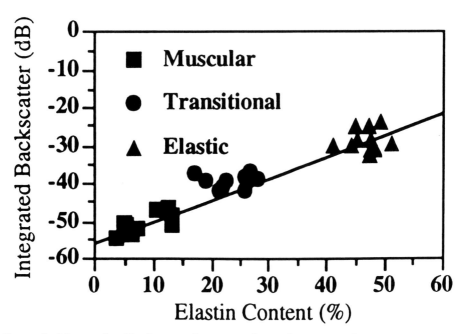

Figure 2. Magnitude of backscatter from normal vascular tissue reflects collagen and elastin content. (With permission, from reference 13)

B. Aortic Aneurysms

Further insights into the physical determinants responsible for the interaction of high frequency ultrasound with arterial tissue are provided by examining the effects of disruption of the collagen and elastin matrix in aortic aneurysms. Aneurysmal dilation of the aorta with subsequent rupture or dissection is a frequent occurrence in patients with Marfan syndrome and the major cause for morbidity. These complications are related to the altered composition and structure of the aortic media, in particular its elastin components. We measured integrated backscatter and anisotropy of backscatter of ultrasound from specimens of aorta from patients with Marfan syndrome undergoing aortic root replacement and compared these values with those from aortic specimens of patients without clinical aortic pathology.

Aortic tissue was obtained at the time of surgery from 11 patients with the Marfan syndrome undergoing repair of an aortic aneurysm or dissection. Normal tissue was obtained at the time of autopsy from 8 patients without evidence of aortic disease. Ultrasonic interrogation was performed at 50 MHZ and integrated backscatter was computed for each specimen. The collagen content of each specimen was determined with a hydroxyproline assay. Marfan aortas exhibited less backscatter than did normal aortas (-40.9 ± 2.9 dB for Marfan vs -32.6 ± 2.2 dB for normals, p<0.0001). No significant difference in collagen concentration was observed between normal and Marfan aorta (262.7 ± 52.7 mg/gm tissue for normals versus 282.4 ± 41.8 mg/gm tissue for Marfan, p=0.42), despite the large difference in backscatter.

Figure 3 shows that aortic segments from these patients manifested a significant decrease in integrated backscatter as compared with normal aorta (approximately 8 dB, or a greater than 6-fold decrease in scattering), despite the presence of similar concentrations of collagen. Histologic analysis revealed striking decrease in both the amount and organization of the elastin in the aortic aneurysm segments from patients with Marfan syndrome as compared with normal aorta. Normal aorta was characterized by well formed elastin fibers arranged in a lamellar pattern. The media from aneurysms in Marfan aorta exhibited a profound decrease in elastin content which was associated with loss of the highly aligned and ordered lamellar arrangement.   Prominent amounts of collagen were present, sometimes in extensive scar-like regions that were interspersed among cystic areas of proteoglycan, but did not appear to be as well aligned overall as in normal arteries.

of proteoglycan, but did not appear to be as well aligned overall as in normal arteries. Therefore, we hypothesize that the *organization* of elastic matrix fibers represents a critical determinant of scattering behavior for arteries at these frequencies.

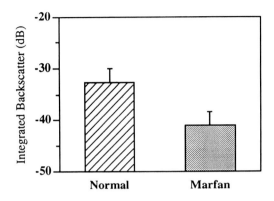

Figure 3: Integrated backscatter from Marfan vs normal aorta (With permission, from reference 13)

To elucidate further the dependence of scattering on tissue organization, the magnitude of ultrasonic anisotropy of backscatter for each tissue type was determined as an index of the three dimensional structure of the vessel matrix (see Figure 4). Vessels were sectioned transversely for insonification perpendicular to circumferentially oriented fibers and longitudinally for insonification parallel to fibers. The magnitude of ultrasonic anisotropy differed dramatically between the two tissue types. Backscatter from normal aorta decreased substantially when the media was insonified parallel as compared with perpendicular to the principal axis of the elastin fibers, whereas Marfan aorta exhibited a much smaller directional dependence of scattering. Normal aortas manifested nearly 12 dB greater ultrasonic anisotropy of integrated backscatter than did Marfan aortas (24.1 ± 3.7 dB for normal versus 12.4 ± 3.3 dB for Marfan, p<0.0001), which is indicative of the profound extent of matrix disorganization in Marfan syndrome. The reduction in the ultrasonic anisotropy of Marfan tissue suggests a marked disorganization of the three dimensional architecture of these aortas and supports the contention that tissue architecture is an important determinant of scattering behavior.

178   S. A. Wickline, et al

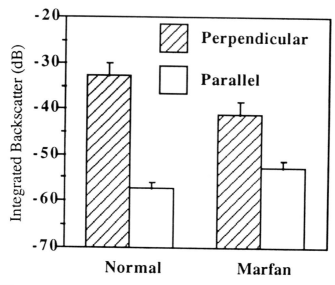

Figure 4 Ultrasonic anisotropy of backscatter for Marfan versus normal aorta (With permission, from reference 13)

The "apparent frequency dependence" of backscatter also can be calculated to provide a clinically applicable index of the frequency content of ultrasound scattered from vascular tissue, as previously reported by Wickline et al for myocardium.[15] The apparent frequency dependence of backscatter was computed as the exponent of a power law relationship between the backscatter transfer function (B(f)) and frequency (f), where $|B(f)|^2 = af^n$, and n is the slope of the line fit for a log-log plot of the backscatter vs frequency.[16] The backscatter values were not compensated for either attenuation or frequency dependent beam volume effects in this case, so that the value for n includes these effects. The slope of the log-log plot for Marfan versus normal aortic tissue differs substantially for perpendicular insonification, but not for parallel insonification. Furthermore, a modest anisotropy of frequency dependence of scattering differentiates Marfan from normal tissue, because there is essentially no difference in the slopes of these plots for perpendicular versus parallel insonification for Marfan but a significant difference in these slopes for normal aortic tissue.

The structural alterations that comprise a loss of well organized elastic tissue lamellae, the dissolution of elastin fibers, the presence of cystic medial necrosis and replacement of matrix materials with large pools of mucopolysaccharide are directly correlated with the loss of anisotropy of frequency dependence of backscatter. These data show that high frequency ultrasonic tissue characterization sensitively detects changes in vessel wall composition and organization which occur in the aorta of patients with aneurysms associated with Marfan syndrome. We have recently determined that aneurysms associated with hypertension and atherosclerotic disease also manifest similar findings and similar histological characteristics. Thus, high frequency ultrasonic tissue characterization may be useful for quantification of abnormalities of vessel wall composition, architecture, and material properties. Although tissue characterization may not differentiate among the various causes of aneurysms, the ability to sensitively detect the physiologic effects of alterations in physical properties and the compromise in vascular structure responsible for early material fatigue could be very important for early diagnosis and followup of patients with these conditions.

C. Atherosclerosis

Recent data indicate that the biological activity of lesions depends on their physical composition and organization. Studies of plaque regression in patients treated with lipid lowering agents have demonstrated that the principal effect of reducing serum cholesterol is to reduce the frequency of acute events such as angina, infarction, heart failure, and bypass surgery. Concomitant with the reduction in clinical events, plaque growth is significantly decelerated. The main outcome is lesion stabilization. Previous pathological studies have demonstrated that lesions with fatty cores covered by fibrous caps appear to be susceptible to rupture and thrombosis due to the concentration of excess stress and strain at the shoulder regions of the caps.[17,18] The presence of tissue macrophages, which can express proteasescapable of digesting the plaque caps at these high stress points, in concert with shear stress imposed by pulsatile flow, establishes the conditions sufficient for plaque rupture. Fibrous lesions are considered to be far more stable and less likely to rupture based on finite element modeling of lesion mechanical properties, which indicate lower and more homogeneous distributions of stress throughout these types of lesions.[19,20] Although it may appear somewhat paradoxical, less severe lesions in the range of 50% stenosis appear to be the most prone to rupture, based on their more fatty composition.

We have shown that high frequency, high resolution ultrasound can quantitatively differentiate between fatty and fibrous plaques.[21] Delineation of the "regression" of atherosclerotic lesions was performed by detecting a change in their composition from fatty to fibrous types induced by alterations in dietary regimen. One group of New Zealand white rabbits was fed a 2% cholesterol diet for 3 months to promote the development of fatty, foam cell rich lesions in the aorta. Another group was fed a similar diet for 3 months, followed by a standard diet for 3 additional months to promote the development of fibrous intimal lesions. Segments of aortas were excised and backscattered radio-frequency data were acquired from 400 to 600 independent sites in each specimen with an acoustic microscope operated at 50 MHZ. Control data were provided by measuring backscatter from adjacent portions of the aortas devoid of lesions. Histologic and immunocytochemical analysis of the fatty lesions confirmed the presence of massive numbers of fat filled foam cells in raised intimal lesions. In contrast, the fibrous intimal lesions comprised smooth muscle cells and abundant connective tissue with little appreciable lipid.

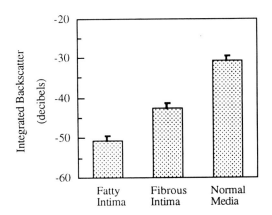

Figure 5: Integrated backscatter from fatty and fibrous intima, and from normal rabbit aorta. (With permission, from reference 13).

Figure 5 shows that backscatter from normal aortic segments (media) (-30.7 ± 1.0 dB) was ≈ 10-fold greater than that from fibrous intimal lesions (-42.4 ± 1.0 dB; $p < 0.05$), which in turn was ≈ 10-fold greater than that from fatty intimal lesions (-50.6 ± 0.7 dB; $p < 0.05$). Values for integrated backscatter from the media of each tissue type were approximately equal (-30.0±1.7 vs -30.7±1.6 vs -33.4±0.8 dB, p = NS for normal vs fibrous vs fatty, respectively). The intimal lesion dimensions in the two groups were approximately equal despite the profound change in physical composition. Removal from the high fat diet lead to evolution of the fatty lesions to a more fibrous, scar tissue-like composition, which is the type of lesion that is clinically more stable (see above). Thus, quantitative ultrasonic tissue characterization sensitively differentiates between fibrous and fatty atherosclerotic plaque and normal tissue in the presence of experimental diet induced atherosclerosis. These results suggest that alterations in dietary regimens may elicit changes in the composition of vascular plaques that are detectable with quantitative ultrasound. The ability to perform these measurements in patients with intravascular ultrasound might provide a useful diagnostic tool for defining the biological activity of potentially dangerous lesions, which now are typically classified as only mild to moderately severe (i.e., ~50% stenosis) by conventional angiography.

III. Tissue Characterization With Intravascular Ultrasound

Wilson et al have recently proposed that "attenuation-slope mapping" with intravascular ultrasound can differentiate among selected lesion types.[22] The measurement of attenuation reflects the reduction in intensity of transmitted ultrasound and is measured in dB/cm. The slope of attenuation represents the dependence of attenuation on frequency and is measured in dB/cm-MHZ. The attenuation slope can be mapped by computing the power spectra from sequential gated segments of rf backscattered from tissue and plotting the signal loss per unit tissue length as a function of distance an frequency. These data can then be used to construct parametric images of vascular tissues. Wilson et al observed that the attenuation slopes of degenerative and calcified plaques exceeded those of normal arteries and those with fibrous plaques. However, the technique may be susceptible to errors derived from heterogeneity of lesion composition, which may cause alterations in the intrinsic scattering behavior of components of lesions that may appear as altered attenuation. Other methods for computing attenuation in vessels have been proposed and tested by Bergers' group and include multi-narrowband and autoregressive spectral analysis techniques.[23]

We have recently developed a technique for providing an accurate reference reflector standard (or near perfect reflector) that is critical for determination of the backscatter transfer function.[24]   A new method of signal calibration also has been developed. This method is based on the classic substitution technique by using a steel reflector as a perfect reference reflector for comparison with the rf signal from the vascular tissue. Unfortunately, some intravascular ultrasound catheter transducers are constructed in a manner which precludes easy alignment for assessment of perpendicular scattering (eg., the Boston Scientific transducer is forward looking by nominally 15 degrees). Rather than designing an adjustable mechanism to allow proper alignment of the reflector, our approach has been to design a reference reflector that would remove the angle dependence of a reference signal. Figure 6 demonstrates this approach. The catheter is placed in the cylinder, inside a guide tube with a physical window positioned to allow imaging only from the center of the cylinder. The inner surface has been honed to a precision surface finish and provides a nearly perfect reflector for ultrasonic scattering. The proposed reference cylinder calibration system can then be used to deconvolve the transducer dependent effects of the backscattered power. An example of the reference rf spectrum and its FFT are shown in Figure 7.

In preliminary experiments, we have demonstrated the ability of quantitative intravascular ultrasound to sensitively detect and quantify the enhancement of reflectivity of blood clots after the application of a novel site-targeted emulsion-based ultrasonic contrast agent recently developed in our laboratory.[25] This problem was chosen because prior work in our laboratory with this contrast agent has demonstrated a strong enhancement of acoustic scattering. Visually, the ultrasonic reflectivity of treated thrombi was markedly enhanced by the addition of the contrast agent. A quantitative difference in scattering power of 5.6 dB was observed with the use of the intravascular ultrasound approach indicating an 3.6 fold increase in backscatter from labelled clots.   This experiment successfully demonstrates the feasibility of obtaining quantitative intravascular ultrasonic data.

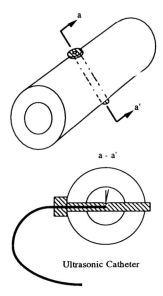

Figure 6:Calibration reference cylinder. (With permission from reference 24)

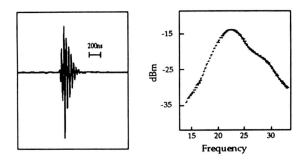

Figure 7: Unprocessed rf signal (left) and magnitude of FFT (right). (With permission, from reference 24)

IV. Clinical Use Of Quantitative Tissue Characterization With Intravascular Ultrasound

Absolute calibration of backscatter data remains a challenge. Issues of spatial resolution, geometrical distortion, diffraction and attenuation compensation, system characterization, transducer variability and robust reference standards need to be addressed.[26,27] If the true difference between purely fatty and fibrous lesions is only 10 dB as suggested by our rabbit data (see above), then the ability to clinically measure small differences in scattering from lesions with mixtures of these characteristics will require care. Furthermore, because coronary artery disease is a diffuse process, the use of adjacent "normal" segments for relative comparisons with the scattering behavior from stenotic lesions may not be justifiable. If intravascular ultrasound is to be used for detection of plaque regression, or change in composition that results in lesion stabilization, it is possible that the precision of backscatter measurements will have to be on the order of 5 dB or less to detect such changes. The manufacturing specifications for catheter performance should accommodate these considerations.

Several physiologic features of the interaction of ultrasound with vascular tissue require consideration. The angle dependence of backscatter and attenuation, or anisotropy, will affect quantitative ultrasonic indexes. Some imaging catheters are even canted to look forward to a certain extent and anisotropy could produce different measurements of scattering behavior for similar vessel morphologies in catheters designed to look forward as compared with those designed to look orthogonal to the vessel wall. Excessive tissue calcification can prevent penetration of sound and limit the ability of intravascular ultrasound to fully characterize lesion composition and morphology. Scattering from red blood cells might also affect quantitative measurements depending on local blood velocity and aggregation of cells, which can increase scattering.[28]

The ultrasonic and mechanical properties of the imaging system also require consideration. Catheter manipulation is generally not as facile as with standard angioplasty balloons due to the necessity of incorporation of a rotating cable in the mechanical systems, which increases the diameter. Lateral resolution may deteriorate with increasing distance from the vessel wall.[29] Better resolution with the use of beam focusing and higher frequencies might improve the ability to characterize potentially unstable lesions, for example those with weaknesses in the thin fibrous cap overlying fatty lesions, as proposed by Lee et al.[20]

From an operational perspective, the procedure is still invasive, and adds time and additional intraarterial manipulation to the catheterization procedure. More important however is the increased expense of the procedure with the addition of intravascular ultrasound. In a patient care environment with fee capitation, the justification for use of expensive therapies such as angioplasty, atherectomy, and intravascular ultrasound will depend on their ability to improve patient outcomes in terms of reduced procedural risk, morbidity, overall mortality, cost, and improved quality of life. It is abundantly clear that lesion composition is key for their biological behavior. Characterization of lesion composition as a guide to prognosis and selection of therapy may provide one significant justification for intravascular ultrasound in a clinical environment, as compared with its use simply as a better gold standard than conventional angiography for determining lesion severity.

V.   Tissue Characterization With Transcutaneous Ultrasound

The application of tissue characterization methods for analysis of ultrasonic backscatter from peripheral and carotid arteries has been modest to date. Most efforts have dealt with the need to delineate unstable plaque in the carotid artery system due to the high morbidity and mortality associated with stroke. Many publications have utilized semiquantitative videodensitometric assessment of plaque characteristics based on routine B-mode images to correlate morphologic features with symptoms such as transient ischemic attacks (TIA). For example, Steinke et al reported that the risk of stroke was greater for heterogeneous and irregular plaques than for those that were smooth and homogeneously echogenic.[30] These heterogeneous plaques contain clot, fibrosis, intraplaque hemorrhage, and irregular calcification. Iannuzzi recently showed that "low lesion reflectivity" was correlated with a recent history of TIA, as were irregular plaques.[31]

The European Carotid Plaque Study also correlated the B-mode appearance of plaques with histologic data from endarterectomy specimens.[32] A subjective grading scale of 1-3 for lesion "echogenicity" was employed. Soft tissue comprised: hemorrhage, lipid, and other "soft constituents" (sic), and calcification and fibrous tissue were classified separately. In general, reduced echogenicity was related to the presence of "soft" components, although the range for diagnosis of "soft" components was quite restricted (20-28%) across the categorical values for echogenicity (value: 1, 2, or 3). In fact, many researchers have opined that the ability of B-mode ultrasound to reliably identify specific plaque components has not yet been established.

A recent paper by Hatsukamai et al from Seattle questions the utility of characterizing components of carotid artery lesions themselves based on the use of traditional B--mode imaging methods.[33] These investigators performed histologic examination of serially sectioned carotid endarterectomy specimens from 43 patients and observed no difference between symptomatic and asymptomatic patients with respect to the presence of lesion fibrosis, intraplaque hemorrhage, lipid core volume, volume of necrosis, or calcification. They concluded that identification of other features of the plaques not routinely visualized by B-mode imaging methods might be more useful for classification., such as the thickness of the fibrous cap overlying the plaque, or the surface morphology (e.g., erosions, thrombosis, etc.). In this regard, it is significant that site targeted imaging of molecular constituents of plaques (see above) such as cross-linked fibrin in microscopic thrombi may permit more accurate delineation of those lesions prone to untoward clinical events (see Figure 8). Additional recent work by Sigel's group supports this hypothesis and indicates that thrombus associated with unstable lesions in carotid artery plaques may be amenable to characterization with the use of a selected combination of backscatter indexes based on spectral analysis methods.[34]

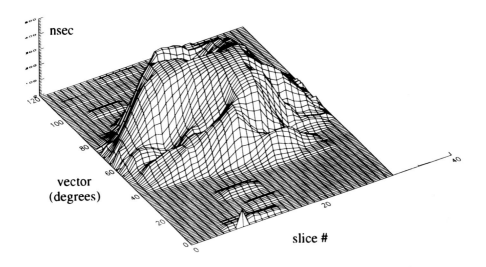

Figure 8: Topographic depiction of morphology of experimental thrombus after application of site targeted ultrasound contrast agent, derived from peak detection of backscatter from thrombus surface in a pseudo three dimensional representation.

References

1. Gussenhoven EJ, Essed CE, Lancee CT, Mastik F, Frietman P, van Egmond FC, Reiber J, Bosch H, van Urk H, Roelandt J, et al.: Arterial wall characteristics determined by intravascular ultrasound imaging: an in vitro study. J Am Coll Cardiol 1989; 14: 947-52
2. Bom N, Slager CJ, Egmond FCv, Lancee CT, Serruys PW: Intra-Arterial Ultrasonic Imaging for Recanalization by Spark Erosion. Ultrasound in Med. & Biol. 1988; 14: 257-26
3. Nishimura RA, Edwards WD, Warnes CA, Reeder GS, Holmes DR, Tajik AJ, Yock PA: Intravascular ultrasound imaging: in vitro validation and pathologic correlation. J Am Coll Cardiol 1990; 16:145-154
4. Picano E, Landini L, Distante A, Sarnelli R, Benassi A, L'Abbate A: Different degrees of atherosclerosis detected by backscattered ultrasound: An in vitro study on fixed human aortic walls. J Clin Ultrasound 1983; 11: 375-379
5. Picano E, Landini L, Lattanzi F, Salvadori M, Benassi A, L'Abbate A: Time domain echo pattern evaluations from normal and atherosclerotic arterial walls: a study in vitro. Circulation 1988; 77:654-659
6. Barzilai B, Saffitz JE, Miller JG, Sobel BE: Quantitative ultrasonic characterization of the nature of atherosclerotic plaques in human aorta. Circ Res 1987; 60:459-463
7. Lockwood GR, Ryan LK, Hunt JW, Foster FS: Measurement of the ultrasonic properties of vascular tissue and blood from 35-65 MHz. Ultrasound Med Biol 1991; 17:653-666
8. Lockwood GR, Ryan LK, Gotlieb AI, Lonn E, Hunt JW, Liu P, Foster FS: In vitro high resolution intravascular imaging in muscular and elastic arteries. J Am Coll Cardiol 1992; 20: 153-160
9. Fitzgerald PJ, St. Goar FG, Connolly AJ, Pinto FJ, Billingham ME, Popp RL, Yock PG: Intravascular ultrasound imaging of coronary arteries. Is three layers the norm? Circulation 1992; 86: 154-8
10. Wickline SA, Barzilai B, Thomas LJI, Saffitz J: Quantification of intimal and medial thickness in excised human coronary arteries with 50 MHz acoustic microscopy. Coronary Artery Disease 1990; 1: 375-381
11. Clark JM, Glagov S: Transmural organization of the arterial media. The lamellar unit revisited. Arteriosclerosis 1985; 5: 19-34
12. de Kroon MGM, van der Wal LF, Gussenhoven WJ, Rijsterborgh H, Bom N: Backscatter directivity and integrated backscatter power of arterial tissue. Int J Card Imaging 1991; 6: 265-275
13. Wickline SA, Miller JG, Recchia D, Sharkey AM, Bridal L, Christy D: Beyond intravascular imaging: Quantitative ultrasonic tissue characterization of vascular pathology Proc IEEE Ultrason Symp 1994; 94CH3468-6: 1589-1597
14. Shepard RK, Miller JG, Wickline SA: Quantification of atherosclerotic plaque composition in cholesterol-fed rabbits with 50 MHz acoustic microscopy. Arteriosclerosis and Thrombosis 1992; 12: 1227- 1234
15. Wickline SA, Verdonk ED, Sobel BE, Miller JG: Identification of human myocardial infarction in vitro based on the frequency dependence of ultrasonic backscatter. J Acoust Soc Am 1992; 91: 3018-3025
16. Sharkey AM, Recchia D, Christy DH, Scott MJ, Wickline SA: Characterization of elastin disruption in Marfan aortopathy with frequency dependent backscatter. J Am Coll Cardiol 1995; Suppl: 290A
17. Davies MJ, Thomas AC: Plaque fissuring- the cause of acute myocardial infarction, sudden ischemic death, and crescendo angina. Br Heart J 1985; 53: 363-373
18. Richardson PD, Davies MJ, Born GVR: Influence of plaque configuration and stress distribution on fissuring of coronary atherosclerotic plaque. Lancet 1989; 941-944
19. Lee RT, Richardson SG, Loree HM, Grodzinsky AJ, Gharib SA, Schoen FJ, Pandian N: Prediction of mechanical properties of human atherosclerotic tissue by high-frequency intravascular ultrasound imaging. An in vitro study. Arteriosclerosis and Thrombosis 1992; 12: 1-5
20. Lee RT: Effects of fibrous cap thickness on peak circumferential stress in model atherosclerotic vessels. Circ Res 1992; 71: 850-8
21. Wickline SA, Shepard RK, Daugherty A: Quantitative ultrasonic characterization of lesion composition and evolution in atherosclerotic rabbit aorta. Arteriosclerosis and Thrombosis 1993; 13: 1543-1550
22. Wilson LS, Neale ML, Talhami HE, Appleberg M: Preliminary results from attenuation slope mapping of plaque using intravascular ultrasound. Ultrasound Med Biol 1994; 20, 529-542
23. Baldeweck T, Laugier P, Herment A, Berger G: Application of autoregressive spectral analysis for ultrasound attenuation estimation: interest in highly attenuation medium. IEEE Trans UFFC 1995; 42: 99-110

24. Christy DH, Wallace KD, Lanza GM, Holland MR, Hall CS, Scott MJ, Cacheris WP, Gaffney PJ, Miller JG, Wickline, SA: Quantitative intravascular ultrasound: Demonstration using a novel site targeted acoustic contrast agent. Proc IEEE Ultrason Symp 1996. (In press).

25. Lanza GM, Wallace KD, Scott MJ, Sheehn CK, Cacheris WP, Christy DH, Sharkey AM, Miller JG Gaffney PJ, Wickline SA: Development and validation of a novel ligand targeted acoustic contrast agent for imaging vascular thrombi. Circulation . (In press).

26. Finet G, Maurincomme E, Tabib A, Crowley RJ, Magnin I, Roriz R, Beaune J, Amiel M: Artifacts in intravascular ultrasound imaging: analysis and implications. Ultrasound in Med Biol 1993; 19, 533-547

27. Hoskins PR, McDicken WN: Techniques for the assessment of imaging characteristics of intravascular ultrasound scanners. Br J Radiol 1994; 67: 695-700

28. Yamada EG, Fitzgerald PJ, Sudhir K, Hargrave VK, Yock PG: Intravascular ultrasound imaging of blood: the effect of hematocrit and flow on backscatter. J Am Soc Echo 1992; 5: 385-92

29. Benkeser PJ, Churchwell AL, Lee C, Abouelnasr DM: Resolution limitations in intravascular ultrasound imaging. J Am Soc Echo 1993; 6: 158-65.

30. Steinke W, Hennerici M, Rautenberg W: Symptomatic and asymptomatic carotid high grade stenosis in Doppler color flow imaging. Neurology 1992; 42: 131-138.

31. Iannuzzi A, Wilcosky T, Mercuri M, Rubba P, Bryan FA, Bond G: Ultrasonographic correlates of carotid atherosclerosis in transient ischemic attack and stroke. Stroke 1995; 26: 614-619.

32. European Carotid Plaque Study Group: Carotid artery plaque composition- -relationship to clinical presentation and ultrasound B-mode imaging. Eur J Vasc Surg 1995; 10: 23-30.

33. Hatsukami TS, Ferguson MS, Beach KW, Gordon D, Detmer P, Burns D, Alpers C, Strandness E: Carotid plaque morphology and clinical events. Stroke 1997; 28: 95-100.

34. Noritomi T, Sigel B, Gahtan V, Swami V, Justin J, Feleppa E, Shirouzu K: In vivo detection of carotid plaque thrombus by ultrasound tissue characterization. J Ultrasound Med 1997; 16: 107-111.

THE IMAGE PROCESSING LABORATORY

David D. McPherson, M.D.

Northwestern University Medical School
Chicago, Illinois   U.S.A.

Contents

I. INTRODUCTION

Vascular ultrasound is a technique that has the ability to characterize the arterial bed and provide specific information concerning the pathophysiologic effects of atherosclerosis. This would include the true geometric structure of the atheroma, surface features including ulcerations, internal plaque characteristics, the degree of vascular remodeling, and the determination of flow characteristics within the vascular bed.

Imaging processing is the use of digital computers to process and analyze medical images. The purpose of this chapter is to describe some basic concepts of image processing and how it can be used to extract additional information from vascular ultrasound. This includes image digitization, storage and display. Processing of images including enhancement and edge detection techniques will then be described followed by variability of vascular ultrasound data collection. Next follows a brief review of three-dimensional vascular reconstruction, the use of acoustic properties to characterize plaque components and the novel uses of ultrasound in atheroma evaluation. As some topics have been described in more detail by the previous authors, this chapter will focus upon image processing techniques for the other processing techniques. Taken together, with the chapters on vascular mechanics and ultrasound characterization of plaque components, this should give the reader a better appreciation of how cardiovascular ultrasound image processing techniques can be used for atheroma evaluation.

II. BASIC CONCEPTS OF IMAGE PROCESSING

Medical ultrasound is the use of high frequency sound waves to record structure and function of biologic tissue. Ultrasound waves tend to be of relatively low energy and long wavelength. Following the emission of sound energy from a transducer, the energy is then reflected to some extent back towards the transducer, which also acts as a receiver and this information is then recorded and displayed on a screen. When ultrasound is sent into a tissue, it interacts with the tissue by attenuating or slowing some of the sound energy as it passes through the tissue, reflecting some of the sound energy back from the tissue; and changing the direction of the acoustic energy as it proceeds through the tissue (refraction). Attenuation is the overall loss of wave amplitude as the propagating sound wave goes through the underlying tissue. The factors that affect attenuation include: scattering by small targets which disperse the wave in many directions; mode conversion which is conversion of ultrasound into different wavelengths as the energy hits large specular targets (i.e. bone); and absorption which is the conversion of wave energy to heat. Reflection is the amount of the sound wave that is sent back to the underlying source. The amount of reflected energy depends on the difference in impedance between two tissue interfaces. Interfaces or materials which have high differences in energy transmission, such as blood and the arterial wall, reflect much more energy back to the transducer than do the various components of the arterial wall itself. Refraction is the change in propagation or forward transmission of a beam as it goes through two interfaces. Refraction of ultrasound is quite great if the sound energy must pass through interfaces of large impedance mismatch, such as blood and the arterial wall (1).

It is not surprising therefore, that reflected ultrasound energy is large from near field structures between interfaces of high impedance mismatch such as the arterial wall and blood versus smaller reflections coming back from components within the arterial wall, especially in the far field.

Additionally, the wavelength of ultrasound in biologic tissue (which is a function of the crystal frequency) determines the frequency of occurrence of a waveform at an interface and thus the amount of reflection of acoustic energy at that interface. The smaller the wavelength, the greater the number of reflections from an interface within the imaging plane. Table 1 describes the approximate wavelength of ultrasound energy for crystal frequencies.

Table 1*

Ultrasound Frequency MHZ	Wavelength (mm)
2.5	0.616
3.5	0.440
5.0	0.308
7.5	0.205
10.0	0.154
12.0	0.128

* Assumes ultrasound propagation velocity of 1540 m/sec for biologic soft tissue.(2)

The use of ultrasound processing techniques can offset some of these known physical properties of ultrasound in biologic tissues. Ultrasound data that returns to the transducer is displayed in a two-dimensional format where every pixel or picture element identifies a certain amount of returning ultrasound energy. The grade or intensity of each pixel is directly proportional to the returning ultrasound energy. Each ultrasound unit has built in signal image modification features (hardware and software) that can provide some processing of the ultrasound information before it is displayed on the screen. These modification features are known in engineering jargon as "curves". Many of these "curves" increase the intensity of the far field reflections, realizing that they are weaker than those from the near field structures. These enhancement features may be linear, logarithmic or variable depending on the curve that it used. In addition to signal modification curves, ultrasound energy can be further modified by adjusting the contrast and brightness on the image screen itself. Therefore, there are a multitude of factors that go together to form a two-dimensional image from the true ultrasound information that is received, the pre-processing that occurs prior to display on the screen and post-processing or image enhancement that occurs after display on the screen. These factors must all be taken into account when evaluating a vascular ultrasound image (3).

A. Image Digitization, Display and Storage

With all diagnostic images come the process of digitization (4). Digitization is essentially, dividing an image into a grid or matrix of discreet positions or pixels. Each position is located by its X and Y coordinates and each pixel position, has attributes of the measured image (sampled) and is assigned a discreet value (quantitized). An ultrasound imaging attribute of interest is the local echo amplitude and is displayed as the grey level. Thus, the digitized ultrasound image can be described as a matrix of pixels, each pixel having a discreet grey level or echo amplitude. Commonly, vascular ultrasound images are displayed in a 512 x 512 pixel matrix. Additionally, depending on the computer storage system, each pixel can be quantitated into a number of grey levels; or amplitudes. In a 4 byte unit there can be 16 grey levels; a 6 byte unit, 64 grey levels; or an 8 byte unit, 256 grade levels for each pixel intensity. Although the human eye can discern fewer than a hundred shades of grey, depending on lighting conditions or for quantitation purposes, a larger number of grey levels may be necessary.

To display an ultrasound image, a video monitor is generally used. A video monitor is a display device in which the horizontal lines are displayed one after another from the top to the bottom of the screen. Following scan conversion, each pixel is displayed on the video monitor with an intensity corresponding to the value of the pixel or the ultrasound amplitude. This relationship between the local ultrasound amplitude and the displayed intensity is generally not linear. This is because the received echo signal as stated above, undergoes non-linear amplification before scan conversion and that the video monitors generally have a display range of only 20 dB. The dynamic range of the unprocessed ultrasound signal may approach 100 dB and therefore a large amount of non-linear compression of the ultrasound signal amplitude occurs prior to digitization and display. Thus, the displayed ultrasound intensity bears a very complex relationship to the actual local echo amplitude (5).

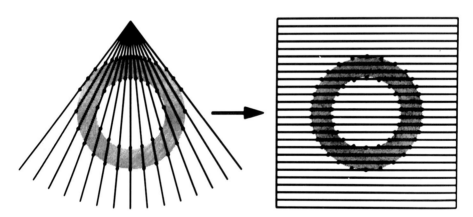

Figure 1. This figure displays how data acquired in polar coordinates must be displayed on a screen in rectangular coordinates. On the right is the conversion of specular reflectors from polar co-ordinates to rectangular co-ordinates with alteration of data for display on the screen. [Reprinted from McPherson, Echocardiography, A Journal of Cardiovascular Ultrasound and Allied Technology 1991; 8:80, with permission]

A digitized image must also be stored. The data is commonly stored onto videotape. However, videotape storage, even with super resolution video fidelity, is hampered by two factors. The first is degradation of image quality that occurs when image data is recorded onto videotape. This is especially noticeable when viewing images in the stop frame mode. The second is the relatively poor temporal stability of the playback mechanism video recorder. This again is most apparent when viewing stop frame images. An alternative approach is to store the image data in digital format within the computer or scanner itself. Although digital storage can provide a much higher resolution of image reproduction, there is an inherent problem between the collection of ultrasound data which is collected in polar coordinates (generally 112-128 radial scan lines each sampled at 400-500 points), and displayed in rectangular coordinates where each scan line lies along the Y axis (see Figure 1 above). A rectangular coordinate pixel display is necessary for display on a regular monitor. The process of conversion of ultrasound image data from a polar to rectangle coordinates adds further variability within the image itself that must be accounted for when analyzing images in digital format (6,7).

B. Processing of Images

B1.   Image Enhancement

Given this complex relationship of an ultrasound image, it is not surprising that what is displayed often requires some degree of image manipulation to be: a) visually pleasing and b) provide the most sophisticated data to appreciate specific image features. Image enhancement is the application of one or more processing steps to an image for the purpose of improving the quality of an image by reducing noise, or in some fashion making the image easier to appreciate (8).

The first image enhancement technique is image smoothing which is used to make portions of ultrasound images similar to their neighbors. This tends to be an averaging technique. There are different types of image smoothing techniques. The most straight forward approach-spatial smoothing - is to replace each pixel with the average of the values of the pixels in its immediate surrounding neighborhood. Thus, each pixel would be replaced by a weighted average of the pixels surrounding it. Spatial smoothing also occurs when an image is processed prior to display. This may occur during the scan conversion process where the data is converted from polar format to a rectangular coordinates where it is necessary to approximate or "fill in" pixels with positions in the rectangular format that fall between digitized points on the origin scan lines. Additionally, images can be spatially smoothed over time. This processing technique identifies the pixels with corresponding X and Y locations in each subsequent image and averages the pixels to produce a time smoothed image without degradation or spatial blurring. This procedure is predicted upon the assumption that the only difference between several sequential images is the amount of noise in the particular image. The problem with spatial smoothing is that if motion has occurred, pixels from different locations within the vascular structure will be averaged, producing undesirable blurring.

Contrast enhancement is another image enhancement technique that makes some image features more visually apparent. A form of contrast enhancement - background image subtraction - subtracts a fixed grey level from the value of all the pixels in the image. This may be arbitrary or may represent some knowledge of the grey levels within the image by use of a gray level histogram. The histogram identifies the relative number of pixels with various grey levels within an image and by changing the histogram, one can change the relative proportion of various grey levels within the image. An example would be to make the histogram more uniform giving a uniform occurrence of all levels of grey within the image. This would have the effect of increasing the number of pixels with intermediate grey levels and is referred to as histogram equalization (8).

Another less commonly used histogram enhancement technique is referred to as histogram hyperbolization (9). This technique attempts to distribute the "perceived" brightness of pixels uniformly.

These and other contrast enhancement procedures can be performed on-line or off-line, using digital computers. Some edge detection techniques described below use contrast enhancement techniques to make borders within an ultrasound image stronger or weaker.

B2. Edge Detection

Edge detection techniques are techniques that allow large specular interfaces or borders to be more easily and consistently defined. These computer processing techniques consist of four basic steps. The first is image preprocessing or enhancement, the second is application of an edge detection operator to the image, followed by a decision as to which pixels are probable edge pixels, the third is deletion or thinning of extraneous or isolated edge pixels and the fourth is filling in gaps to form continuous borders.

Preprocessing, again, enhances the images and is used to reduce image noise and improve the accuracy of subsequent edge detection techniques. These include contrast enhancement techniques such as histogram equalization.

Edge detection operator techniques look at the probability that an intensity gradient between various pixels best describes an edge. The simplest type of edge operator technique is that of thresholding in which a certain value (defined as a change in the grey level from one pixel to another) is arbitrarily defined as the border. A more sophisticated edge detection operator looks at the changes or gradients across an image and identifies the slope of the changes or an arbitrary change in the slope as the edge (10).

Another edge detection operator which has been increasingly used, is that in which the operator manually identifies the border in one image set. Subsequently, using the gradients that have been manually identified, the computer searches previous or future images, and using gradients or thresholds in similar positions and space, identifies borders. By adding the manual input of one image, the computer does much less searching or calculation of gradient thresholds within an image. A more novel edge detection operator is to take an image processing technique that mathematically matches expected morphology (shape and structure in an image). Klinger et al, (11) have used this mathematically expected morphology to identify image borders. Feng et al, (12) have enhanced this by introducing a fuzzy set theory. This technique starts with a known border recognition program and introduces some degree of fuzziness into the program, such that when the image is evaluated by the border recognition package, fuzziness is expected prior to contour definition. This method is excellent for ultrasound images as some degree of fuzziness is present in all images.

In our own laboratory, we have expanded on the above edge detection logic by using a Hough transform border recognition package with some elements of fuzzy theory to identify borders within cine-CT, echocardiographic and intravascular ultrasound image data (13, 14, 15) (Figure 2). This technique shows exciting promise in that it is a novel way to approach acoustic images for border recognition.

The last type of edge detection uses unprocessed radiofrequency (RF) (or some variation of RF) ultrasound data. The RF energy of each scan line is used to identify borders. In this method large RF energy changes identify borders in the 2-D image. This method is good for near field borders between low to high reflected energy structures but due to acoustic ringdown is often not very good for high to low reflected energy structures.

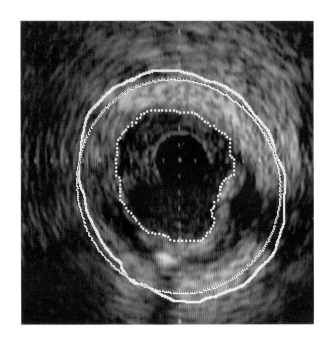

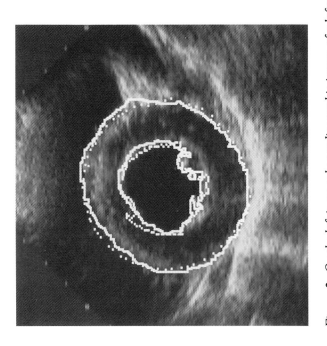

Figure 2. On the left is an echocardiographic image of a left ventricle in cross section and on the right an intravascular ultrasound image of an atherosclerotic artery in cross section. Straight lines represent manually traced (segmented) lumen and outer wall contours. Dotted lines represent computer identified edges. (Figure courtesy of Dr. E. L. Dove).

Following border identification, the third step is an edge thinning or deletion procedure. This is necessary because of the many edges or similarities identified within an acoustic image that may be due to reverberation or acoustic speckle. These sources of noise must be deleted and many "thinning" algorithms can be utilized to eliminate isolated and extraneous edge pixels (16).

The fourth and final step is the filling in of gaps between edges to make the edges continuous within the image. If there is much image preprocessing or the image is smoothed initially, then there are generally very few gaps that require filling. However, if there is little initial smoothing, often a smoothing program must be used at the end to identify continuous borders.

The result of these four steps is that edges are detected within an image that have some relationship to the true geometry of the structure of interest. However, the validity of such edges require extensive in-vitro (bench and autopsy specimen) and in-vivo (animal and patient) testing and validation. Although many of these image processing algorithms for edge detection work in theory, in practice, manual tracing (manual segmentation) of all image borders using constant image processing settings is what is generally performed. Future work will determine whether variations of these new image processing techniques are useful for constant and reproducible evaluation of borders within vascular ultrasound images.

C. Variability within Vascular Ultrasound

There are standard types of ultrasound variability of which every investigator needs to be aware. These include two-point structural resolution, image thickness, pathologic impedance, image enhancement, digitalization, and storage and display methods. Image enhancement, digitalization, storage and display methods have been previously covered.

Two-point structural resolution depends upon the transducer frequency as well as the focus of the transducer crystals. As the frequency of an ultrasound transducer is increased, the waveform decreases and the resultant two-point structural resolution increases. This is at the expense of a decreasing depth of field of the crystal (depth of field = penetration of the ultrasound in tissue). Standard 2.25 - 3.50 MHZ transducers have actual two-point structural resolutions of 0.5-1.0 cm with an imaging depth of up to 30cm. At 7.5 MHZ the resultant two-point structural resolution within the imaging field of the transducer is 0.2-0.3mm; this increases to 0.1-0.2mm using a 12 to 13 MHZ transducer and further to 0.1mm using 20 to 40 MHZ transducers. However, the latter transducers have depths of imaging field only up to 10 mm. The trade off therefore is that although the imaging resolution increases with increasing crystal frequency, the resultant depth of imaging penetration markedly decreases.

Therefore, although increasing the transducer frequency will increase the resolution of vascular structures within an ultrasound image, the penetration of the waveform is markedly reduced. For standard purposes, 7.5 MHZ transducers are used transcutaneously for B-mode imaging of the carotid and ileofemoral beds: 20 to 40 MHZ transducers are used intravascularly for evaluation of peripheral and coronary arteries; and 13 MHz transducers are used for intraoperative vascular scanning at the time of operation.

Another source of variability is that each ultrasound image also has some relative thickness. This thickness is very small if only one crystal is being used for imaging, however, increases dramatically if multiple crystals at fixed spacing distances are used. Intravascular ultrasound, which traditionally uses one crystal, has a smaller slice thickness (0.25 mm at the focal distance 6-10 mm) versus B-mode transcutaneous ultrasound which uses multiple crystals and has larger slice thickness (1 mm at the focal distance).

Pathologic features also cause image variability. Ultrasound principles are generally used for soft tissue in which ultrasound is reflected and penetrates the tissue to varying degrees. However, calcium is the classic example of a pathologic structure that can completely impede the ultrasound penetration. Therefore, calcium causes acoustic shadowing within an image and there is loss of information behind the calcium. Similarly, structures such as calcium can cause acoustic signals at positions of the same depth but altered horizontal position. This phenomenon is known as "side lobe artifact". These and other pathologic features cause variability within images.

Given the marked variability of B-mode and vascular ultrasound images, it is important that all equipment be uniformly standardized and that the same or very similar equipment and processing techniques be used if patients are to be examined at multiple times during interventional trials for true differences to be found. If different equipment is being used at different times to monitor atheroma progression/regression, then it can be easily seen that equipment and image processing related variability may be so large as to mask any true changes that have occurred within the vascular bed.

III. THREE-DIMENSIONAL VASCULAR RECONSTRUCTION

An image processing technique that has wide applicability for use with vascular ultrasound is three-dimensional reconstruction (3DR). Although covered by Vonesh and Chandran, this chapter will deal primarily with image processing and how it is used to perform 3DR.

Steps in Three-Dimensional Reconstruction

To obtain a 3D reconstruction of a vascular ultrasound image, a number of steps must be undertaken. The first step is the connection of the vascular ultrasound probe to a device that allows the identification of the image coordinates of each vascular ultrasound image in space. This can be obtained through either a device attached to the probe that acts as a transmitter or receiver or can be used through methods such as bi-plane angiography which uses another imaging technique to determine the ultrasound image plane's position in space.

Fix PRD in Space over the Vascular Segment

Scan Artery of Interest; Record Images and Location of Each Image in Space

Following determination of the spatial coordinates of each image, the image borders must be identified. Borders can be traced (segmented) automatically via computer algorithms, or traced manually. Border segmentation allows the image to be computer processed. If a large computer memory is available, these images are entered in a 512 x 512 (or similar) pixel matrix allowing full grey scale levels for each pixel. In a system that utilizes less computer processing capabilities, image borders are often traced (manually segmented) and only the information between the images are

Boundary Definition of Lumen and Wall

Image Orientation, 3D Reconstruction

entered in a 512 x 512 (or similar) pixel matrix allowing full grey scale levels for each pixel. In a system that utilizes less computer processing capabilities, image borders are often traced (manually segmented) and only the information between the traced borders is entered into the computer, generally in a black/white; 0/255 format).

Once the image data are entered into the computer and oriented accurately in space, then a second algorithm joins data between individual images. This data generally is the weighted average of the information at similar pixel locations between images. Therefore, if a pixel at location X in image one has a grey scale of 56 and the pixel at the same position in the second image has a grey scale of 28, then the two would be weighted and pixels of 42 would be put between image one and image two at those positions in space that have no image data. It can easily be seen that if images are spaced very closely together, that very little data has to be added to make the 3D reconstruction. If images are quite far away in space, then much data must be added of which most may not be correct.

After all the missing information has been added between the image sets, the vascular segments then must be displayed visually on a screen for viewing. This is generally displayed in pseudo 3D format where a different grey scale shading algorithm is used to provide depth. The image can then be manipulated such that the outer arterial wall is displayed in pseudo 3D, the inner luminal borders displayed, or the layers can be peeled off one at a time at varying depths of field allowing display of the arterial segment at various levels. All of this information is stored within a computer and can be extracted, depending on the requirement. (Examples would be visualization of surface topography- ulcers, craters and thrombi- or visualization of inner plaque components.) There are presently two types of 3D reconstruction techniques available on the market, those for use with intravascular ultrasound data and those used for transcutaneous B-mode ultrasound data.

A. Three-Dimensional Reconstruction of Intravascular Ultrasound Data

High frequency intravascular ultrasound (IVUS) is a technique that allows two-dimensional display of vascular structure in-vivo. It uses intravascular catheters have diameters as small as 1 mm and distally positioned 20-40 MHz transducers. By placing the catheters within the arterial segment to be interrogated, in-vivo imaging of peripheral and coronary arteries can be accomplished producing images with excellent structural definition of lumen and wall (17,18,19). There are, however, technical limitations to the procedure (20). Only single two-dimensional (2D) images are obtained and displayed at any given time. The operator is required to mentally integrate a series of transverse images to determine spatial relationships. As the images are obtained in a plane perpendicular to the long axis of the catheter, direct longitudinal vessel information and relationships are not displayed. The length of lesions and distance between landmarks can only be inferred by movement of the catheter.

To overcome the obstacles of the two-dimensional IVUS imaging, three-dimensional (3D) reconstruction have been generated from these ultrasound data (21,22). This provides longitudinal information. The 3D display format provides a convenient way of displaying the 2D ultrasound data and appears to provide useful information concerning pathology including dissections, post-intervention. These reconstructions do not provide accurate spatial information. The IVUS images are assumed to be parallel tomographic slices which are reconstructed in a stack. Thus, the reconstructed vessels are shown without curves. The distance between landmarks is determined by the time required to traverse the segment with the catheter. With variation of pullback rate, vessel segments may be erroneously displayed and therefore elongated, or shortened. Wiet et al, (23) have demonstrated that linear 3D reconstruction techniques introduce substantial catheter-dependent geometric error in vessels with small radii of curvature. To overcome these obstacles, we and others have developed 3DR techniques that accurately display image data in space (24). Elaborating upon an algorithm described by McKay et al (25), we now use bi-plane fluoroscopy to identify intravascular ultrasound catheter coordinates. The catheter position is used to identify the location of the intravascular ultrasound image data sets. Coordinate positions are identified and referenced to positions documented with a calibration cube. Phantom studies, in-vitro studies and patient studies demonstrate the accuracy of such reconstructions (24). Figure 3 illustrates an angiogram of a spiral phantom on the left with corresponding reconstruction of the spiral phantom by intravascular ultrasound on the right. Note the good demonstration of curves and tortuosity in these reconstruction. Figure 4 illustrates the comparison of actual versus calculated distance, volume and area measurements for the phantom coronary arterial segments using this accurate 3D reconstruction technique. There is good agreement between the actual and calculated measurements. Figure 5 illustrates an angiogram of the left anterior descending coronary artery (left) with the corresponding 3D IVUS reconstruction of the segment (outer arterial wall) to the left. Again, note the good reconstruction throughout the early portion of the curve. Figure 6 illustrates an intravascular ultrasound 3D reconstruction of a segment of a saphenous vein graft with the corresponding angiographic image to the left. On the angiogram S and F point to the start and finish of the reconstruction. The error in the reconstruction identifies vessel movement due to peeling (accordioning) as the catheter is pulled thru the curve of this relatively free floating vascular segment. Other authors have demonstrated the feasibility of other 3D reconstruction techniques for intravascular ultrasound data (26). The potential with these techniques now lies in the relative ability of intravascular ultrasound to identify the vascular segment in 3D and accurately determining atheroma composition and mass within the reconstructed vascular segment.

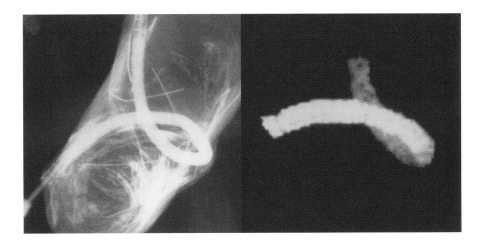

*Figure 3. Angiogram **(left)** and 3D-IVUS reconstruction **(right)** of a spiral phantom. See text for details.*

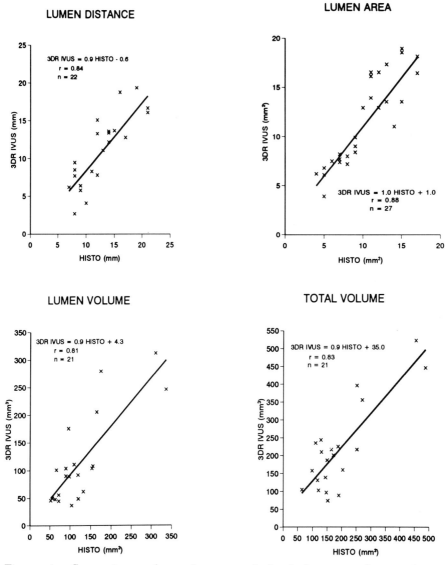

Figure 4. Comparisons of actual verses calculated distance, volume and area measurements using the accurate 2D reconstruction technique.

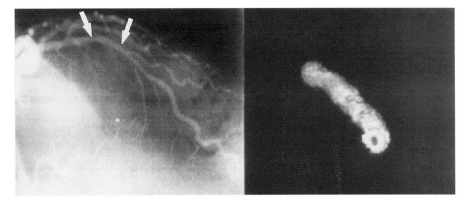

Figure 5. Angiogram (A) and 3D reconstruction (B) of a portion of the left anterior descending coronary artery.

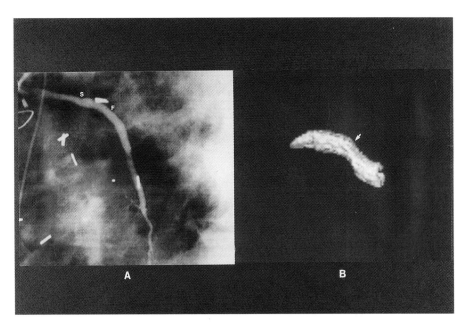

Figure 6. Angiogram (A) and 3D reconstruction (B) of a saphenous vein graft demonstrating a curve caused in the reconstruction due to vessel movement as the catheter is withdrawn through the graft.

B.   Three-Dimensional Reconstruction of Transcutaneous B-Mode Ultrasound Data

Transcutaneous B-mode ultrasound data is an excellent imaging technique that provides high resolution imaging of arterial walls. It allows for detailed imaging of the carotid, ilio-femoral and other superficial arterial beds. For three-dimensional reconstruction, position registration devices for transcutaneous ultrasound transducers have been developed. A device we have developed allows one degree of freedom and documents the pullback speed of the ultrasound data so that smooth image data can be obtained over vascular segments of up to 5 cm. Unlike IVUS, this device and 3DR algorithm does not require the object to be at a fixed position in each image, but rather joins the information on the object depending on where it lies in the image with respect to each of its neighbors. Preliminary results demonstrate the feasibility and accuracy of this technique for evaluation of the carotid (27) and femoral beds (28). Figure 7 illustrates a 3DR of a carotid arterial bifurcation demonstrating an atherosclerotic plaque protruding into the lumen. The outer arterial reconstruction is demonstrated on the left and the inner geometry with the protruding atherosclerotic plaque (arrow) is on the right. In this example, the bifurcation can be nicely demonstrated. Figure 8 illustrates a 3D reconstruction of a femoral artery (left). This outer reconstruction can be manipulated such that the inner luminal geometry is demonstrated (right).

One limitation of linear 3D reconstruction techniques for B-mode ultrasound data, is that only one degree of freedom is available and therefore, two separate pullbacks with data set integration are often required to accurately identify all anatomic components of the carotid or iliofemoral regions.

A new technique that provides a freely moving 3D reconstruction device utilizes a "Flock of Birds" (FOB) position sensing device. This sensor technology (Ascension Technology, Burlington, VT.) has been used in a variety of applications requiring highly accurate, non-restricted determination of 3D position such as robotics, computerized design manufacturing and Virtual Reality. The FOB uses the detected strength of a direct current (DC) magnetic field to sense the geometrical relationship between a magnetic field transmitter-receiver pair. This identifies the X, Y and Z coordinates of each image set with respect to the next image set. Six full degrees of freedom are allowed. Preliminary results using the FOB technology demonstrates it is highly accurate for phantoms and in-

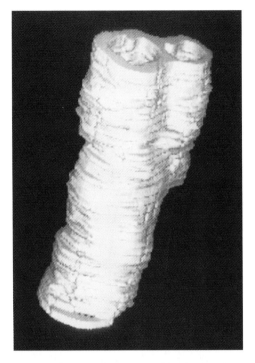

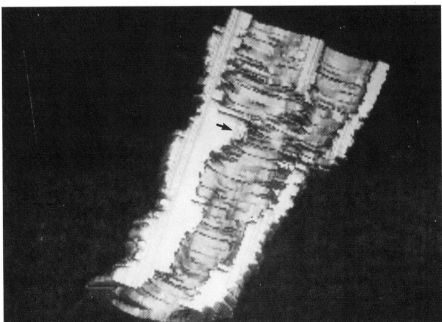

Figure 7. Outer (top) and inner (bottom) 3D reconstruction of a carotid arterial bifurcation.

vitro vascular data (29). Preliminary patient validation is underway. Figure 9 illustrates the FOB attached to a vascular transducer demonstrating its very small compact design. To the right is a 3D reconstruction of an in-vitro vascular segment using this technique.

The techniques of B-mode 3D reconstruction - especially those that allow unrestricted probe movement should accurately identify surface topographic features of the atherosclerotic plaques within the carotid and iliofemoral beds. This information would be invaluable in assessing the geometric structure, atheroma characteristics and atheroma mass for diagnosis and to evaluate changes following intervention.

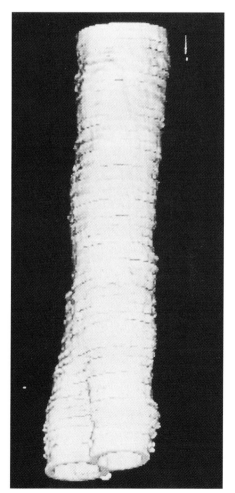 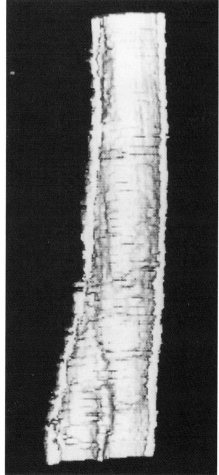

Figure 8. Outer (left) and inner (right) 3D reconstruction of a femoral artery.

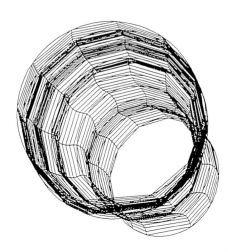

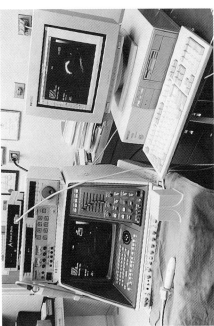

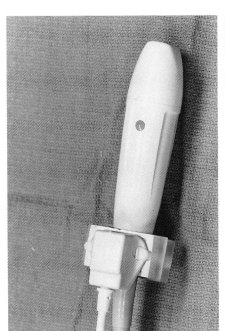

Figure 9. "Flock of Birds" technology for accurate 3DR of B-mode ultrasound data. On the top left is the device attached to an ultrasound transducer. On the bottom left is the equipment setup. On the right is a 3DR using preliminary data generated from this unit.

IV. USE OF ACOUSTIC PROPERTIES TO CHARACTERIZE
PLAQUE COMPONENTS

Much acoustic information obtained at the time of the vascular ultrasound examination is not utilized other than in a very superficial way for visual image analysis. Much of the unused information, concerns the relative intensities or frequencies of data between the specular reflectors. The use of ultrasound to identify various components within a tissue is known as ultrasound tissue characterization. This may be useful for the identification of atherosclerotic plaque components. The chapter by Wickline deals with tissue characterization in detail.

With respect to image processing, the necessary components for tissue characterization are a knowledge of the type of ultrasound, intensity and pattern within the tissue. This information could either be the grey scale level of the ultrasound within a region of interest in a 2D ultrasound image, or the power spectrum or components of the signal using radiofrequency or A-mode ultrasound. Many vascular and intravascular ultrasound transducers have A-mode lines of site which can be obtained from regions of interest within the tissue. Investigators including Barzilai et al, (30) and Ng et al, (31) have looked at the various components of radiofrequency ultrasound signals and found that the energy and waveform patterns can separate calcified from fibrous plaques from normal underlying wall (Figure 10).

These techniques may allow for the determination of early plaque components, plaques with ulcerations and thrombus that are prone to rupture, plaques with large fatty lakes which may be unstable, and plaques with large components of calcium and fibrous tissue which may be quite stable and chronic lending themselves to removal by mechanical interventions.

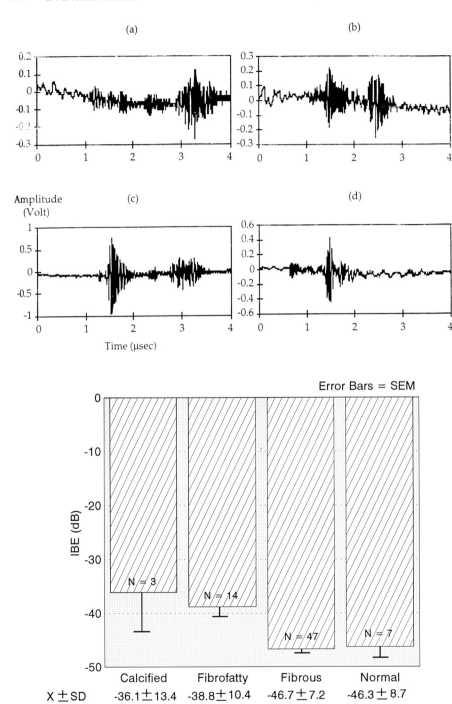

Figure 10 **(Top)**. *Radio-frequency power spectrum for normal wall (a) , fibrous (b), fibro fatty (c) and calcified (d) plaques. 10* **(Bottom)** *Integrated backscatter energy results for these specimens.*

V. NOVEL USES OF ULTRASOUND

A. Liposomes and Other Targetable Agents for Acoustic Plaque Enhancement

Some image processing techniques have great potential for the extraction of further information from vascular ultrasound. The use of target-specific acoustic enhancement agents would highlight components of the altered endothelium or atherosclerotic plaque. One such novel and exciting acoustic enhancement agent is the use of target specific liposomes. Liposomes are vesicles generally less than one micron in diameter made up of various combinations of phospholipids (32). Liposomes are non-toxic and can be injected into different compartments in the body. Liposomes have been developed, using either encapsulated gas (33) or lyophilization (freeze drying)(34) allowing liposomes to be acoustic enhancement agents. Charges between liposomes, multiple layers within the liposomes , and markedly thickened liposomal layers providing great acoustic mismatches are potential explanations for their acoustic highlighting properties.

Liposomes have been formulated so that they can be conjugated to antibodies while retaining their acoustic properties (35). In the early stages of plaque formation, monocytes are recruited to the injured endothelial cells by associated vascular adhesion molecules (VCAM) (36). VCAM are important indicators of activated endothelial cells surrounding the atherosclerotic plaque (37). A second endothelial adhesion molecule, intercellular adhesion molecule - (ICAM-1) has been shown to enhance recruitment of circulatory monocytes near the plaque and vasovasorum (38, 39). Other components within the atheromatous lesion such as fibrin and D-dimers are abundant (40). If conjugated liposomes could be targeted to acoustically enhanced pathologic endothelium of the atherosclerotic plaque, then various components in the plaque in early or more advanced stages of atheroma development could be evaluated. Examples would be plaques rich in fibrin or plaques that are likely to undergo thrombosis and/or plaque rupture. In addition to identifying active plaque morphology, this would lead to better tailoring of medical or interventional therapy.

Other agents have been developed that provide targeted acoustic highlighting. Two such agents undergoing development are perflurorocarbon microemulsions and perfluorobutane - gas filled microspheres (41,42,43). Using ligands that target to fibrin both have been able to enhance thrombi in arterial and veinous beds. The potential uses of these agents would be to highlight plaque characteristics such as fibrin within craters or ulcerations that would predispose to thrombus formation and embolization.

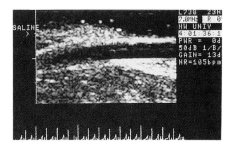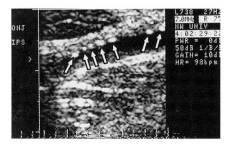

Figure 11. Transvascular ultrasonic images of the left carotid artery in an atherosclerotic miniswine: (Left) prior to injection of liposomes; (Right) following injection of anti-ICAM 1 labeled liposomes with liposomal attachment to the atheroma. (Arrows point to liposomes.)

B.   Forward Viewing Intravascular Ultrasound

Another novel use of vascular ultrasound is the development of forward viewing intravascular ultrasound. Standard IVUS catheters image perpendicular to the long axis of the catheter and can be thought of as side viewing. Transverse images of the vascular structure are obtained lateral to the catheter. Images cannot be obtained forward of the catheter tip. These instruments are unable to provide anatomic information in small vessels, obstructions, or in vessels in which placement of a catheter would create potential problems (such as the carotid arteries). Forward viewing intravascular ultrasound catheters place the imaging transducers at the end of the imaging device and image forward to the transducer. We in conjunction with Boston Scientific Imaging Systems (Sunnyvale, CA), have developed an ultrasound catheter that images ahead of the transducer. It has a 20 MHZ single crystal and can image to a depth of 2 cm, with an axial resolution of 0.12 mm and lateral resolution of 0.23 mm. (11 left).   Figures 11 (middle and right) and 12 illustrate forward-viewing intravascular ultrasound images. Initial in vitro and animal validation studies have demonstrated excellent structural definition using this device (44, 45).

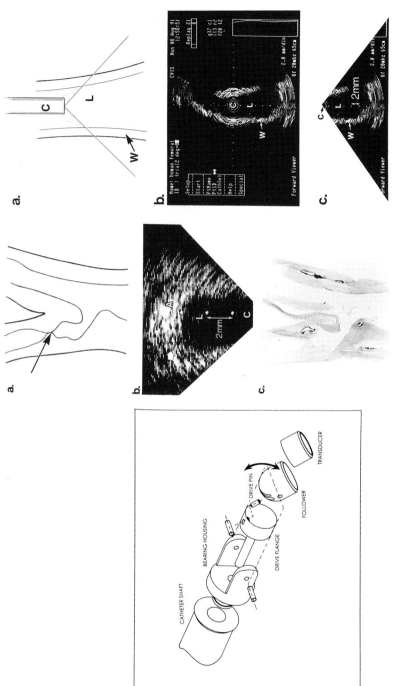

Figure 12. (Left) Schematic of the forward viewing IVUS catheter. (Middle) schematic of an in-vitro canine aorta (a), intravascular ultrasound image (b), and IVUS image with redundant information removed (c). (Right) schematic (a), (IVUS) image (b) and pathologic specimen (c) of occluded carotid artery. C indicates catheter; L, lumen; W, wall. Arrows point to walls; or atheromatous carotid occlusion; calibration marks are 2 mm. (From Evans et al, and the American Heart Association with Permission. Ref. 44).

The use of three-dimensional reconstruction of these forward viewing IVUS data provides a good means of obtaining topographical information.   Ng et al, (46) demonstrated a 3D reconstruction technique using   forward viewing intravascular ultrasound data with excellent structural resolution by taking data obtained for every 5⁰ of rotation of the transducer (Figure 13).

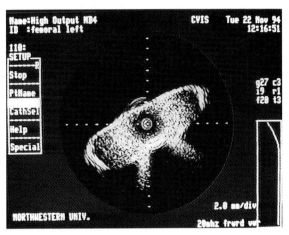

Figure 13.   An in-vivo ultrasound image of a femoral artery   demonstrating the superficial femoral   arterial take off. Calibration   marks are 2 mm. Redundant information has not been removed.

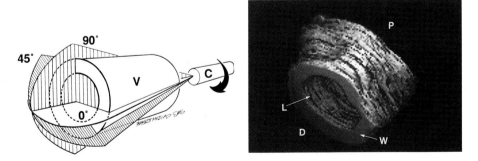

Figure 14.   A schematic of the principle of catheter rotation for forward viewing 3DR (Left). A three-dimensional reconstruction of approximately 1 cm of a canine aortic segment using forward viewing 3DR (Right).   The proximal aorta close to the catheter is located 1 cm away from the transducer. Indentations and distal narrowing are easily noted. P indicates proximal; D, distal; L, lumen; and W, wall. (From Ng et al, and the American Heart Association with permission Ref. 46).

C. Acoustic Emissions to Characterize Plaque Rupture

Another novel use of ultrasound is the evaluation of acoustic emissions to determine morphologic changes within an atherosclerotic plaque.

"As a structure undergoes mechanical alteration, acoustic emissions are generated." This well known phenomenon in materials testing has been used to test the strength of plastics, metal and concrete products. Vonesh et al, was able to demonstrate that acoustic emissions are emitted when a carotid plaque undergoes alterations due to balloon angioplasty (47). This phenomenon occurs when the atherosclerotic plaque is being expanded by the angioplasty catheter and micro and macro fractures are occurring within the plaque, due to angioplasty induced trauma. Using in-vitro pathologic arterial specimens, he was able to demonstrate that both the pattern of and the frequency of these acoustic emissions separate angioplasty induced micro dissections from pathologic macro dissections (48). These acoustic emissions could be used in therapeutic balloon angioplasty to determine the threshold above which major tissue trauma occurs. Figure 15 demonstrates the recording of acoustic emissions during balloon induced angioplasty in one the in-vitro specimens. The arrow points to the increase of the acoustic emissions

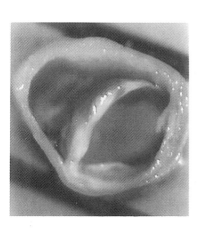
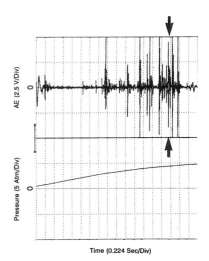

Figure 15. *(Left)* *Atherosclerotic specimen demonstrating dissection information.* *(Right)* *Plot of emissions release vs inflation time demonstrating the release of acoustic emissions with plaque rupture and subsequent dissection. Evaluating the pattern and release of acoustic emissions may allow for determination of optimal plaque fracture.*

during of dissection formation. The novel use of this acoustic emission catheter may allow for better guiding of mechanical intervention, such as balloon angioplasty, in order to minimize procedural complications.

VI. SUMMARY

These and other new ultrasound techniques are expanding the field of vascular ultrasound allowing more information to be extracted from ultrasound signals. This information would allow better diagnostic evaluation of the pathologic features within each vascular bed, better tailoring of interventional therapies (mechanical or pharmacological) and allow more accurate follow-up of the results of interventions to limit or reduce the effects of atheroma.

This chapter has attempted to address some of the fundamental concepts of ultrasound and ultrasound imaging for evaluation of vascular anatomy. In particular it has dealt with some of the basic concepts of image processing including image digitization, new ways of processing ultrasound images and variability within ultrasound image data. Three-dimensional vascular reconstruction is a new and novel way to demonstrate vascular morphology both using intravascular and transcutaneous ultrasound data. Radiofrequency ultrasound techniques have use in the characterization of atherosclerotic plaque components. There are new and novel uses of ultrasound including acoustic plaque enhancement techniques, forward viewing intravascular ultrasound and acoustic emissions to depict plaque rupture. Due to its use and ability to depict the morphologic components of the arterial wall, ultrasound seems to be an excellent technique for following and evaluating atherosclerosis. The next chapter deals with ongoing and potential uses of ultrasound in atheroma regression trials using either presently available ultrasound or ultrasound with newer image processing techniques.

Acknowledgments

I would like to thank *Cynthia Shane* for her expert preparation of this chapter and *Bonnie Kane* for her technical assistance.

References

1. Geiser EA, Oliver LH. Echocardiography: Physics and Instrumentation. In Cardiac Imaging and Image Processing - Collins SM, Skorton DJ (eds). McGraw Hill, 1986; 3-9.
2. Wells PNT. Biomedical Ultrasonics. Academic Press, 1977; 20.
3. Gonzalez RC, Woods R. Digital Imaging Processing. Reading, MA, Addison-Wesley. 1992; 10-16.
4. Thomas JD. Digital image processing. In: Principles and Practice of Echocardiography. 2nd Edition. Weyman AE (ed). Lea and Febiger, 1994; 56-57.
5. White DN. Ultrasound in Medical Diagnosis, Kingston, Ontario, Ultramedicine Press, 1976; 168-170.
6. Aylward PE, Knosp BN, McPherson DD, et al. Two-dimensional echocardiographic image texture analysis. reduction of regional variability using polar co-ordinates. Ultrasonic Imaging, 1985; 7:60-73.
7. McPherson DD, Aylward PE, Knosp BN, et al. Ultrasound characterization of acute myocardial ischemia by polar texture analysis. Ultrasonic Imaging 1987; 8:227-240.
8. Garcia E, Ezekiel A, Levy R, et al.: Automated computer enhancement and analysis of left ventricular two-dimensional echocardiograms. Computers in Cardiology, Long Beach, CA, IEEE Computer Society 1982; 399-402.
9. Frei W. Image enhancement by histogram hyperbolization. Comput Graphics Image Processing 1977; 6:286.
10. Skorton DJ, McNary CA, Child JS, Newton FC, Shah PM. Digital image processing of two-dimensional echocardiograms: identification of the endocardium. Am J Cardiol 1981; 48:479.
11. Klinger JW, Franker TD and Andrews LT. Segmentation of echocardiographic images using mathematical morphology. IEEE Trans. Biomed Eng. 1984; 35:925-933.
12. Feng J, Lin WC, Chen CT. Epicardial boundary detection using fuzzy reasoning. IEEE Trans Med Imaging 1991; 10:187-199.
13. Philip KP, Dove EL, McPherson DD, Gotteiner NL, Stanford W, Chandran KB.. The fuzzy hough transform feature extraction in medical images. IEEE Trans Med Imaging 1994; 13:235-240.
14. Dove EL, Philip KP, Gotteiner NL, Vonesh MJ, et al. A method for automatic edge detection, volume computation and three-dimensional reconstruction of the left ventricle from ultrafast computed tomographic images. Investigative Radiology 1994; 11:945-954.
15. Wiet SP, Sinha R, Greenfield SA, et al. Automatic border detection of intravascular ultrasound. J Am Coll Cardiol 1996; 29:240A.
16. Stefanelli R, Rosenfeld A: Some parallel thinning algorithms for digital pictures. J Assoc Comput Machinery 1971; 18:255.
17. Nissen SE, Grines CL, Gurley JC, et al. Application of a new phased array ultrasound imaging catheter in the assessment of vascular dimensions: A comparison to cineangiography. Circulation 1990; 81:660-666.
18. Tobis JM, Mallery J, Lehman K, et al. Intravascular ultrasound imaging of human coronary arteries in vivo: Analysis of tissue characterization with comparison to in vitrohistological specimens. Circulation 1991; 83:913-926.
19. Yock PG, Johnson EL, David DT. Intravascular ultrasound: Development and clinical potential. Am J Card Imaging 1988; 2:185-193.
20. Roelandt J, di Mario C, Pandian NG. Three-dimensional reconstruction of intracoronary ultrasound images: Rationale, approaches, problems and directions. Circulation 1994; 90:1044-1055.
21. Kitney RI, Moura L, Straughan K. 3D visualization of arterial structures using ultrasound and voxel modelling. Int J Card Imaging 1989; 4:177-185.
22. Rosenfield K, Lorsordo DW, Ramaswamy K, et al. Three-Dimensional reconstruction of human coronary and peripheral arteries from images recorded during two-dimensional intravascular ultrasound examination. Circulation 1991; 84:1938-1956.
23. Wiet SP, Vonesh MJ, Waligora MJ, Kane BJ, McPherson DD. The effect of vascular curvature on three-dimensional reconstruction of intravascular ultrasound images. Ann Biomed Eng 1996; 24:695-701.
24 Evans JL, Ng KH, Wiet SP, et al. Accurate Three-dimensional reconstruction of Intravascular Ultrasound Data: Spatially correct three-dimensional reconstructions. Circulation 1996; 93:567-576.
25. McKay S, Potel MJ, Rubin JM. Graphics methods for tracking three-dimensional heart wall motion. Computers and Biomed Res 1982; 15:455-473.
26. Slager CJ, Laban M, von Birelen C. 'ANGUS': A new approach to three-dimensional reconstruction of geometry and orientation of coronary lumen and plaque by combined use of coronary angiography and IVUS. J Am Coll Cardiol 1995; 25:144A.

27. Vonesh MJ, Mesh C, Ng KH, Blackburn DR, McPherson DD, Yao JST. Three-dimensional reconstruction of the carotid bifurcation with vascular ultrasound using a new position registration device. Circulation 1991; 84:11-22.
28. Hart JP, Vonesh MJ, Durham JR, et al. Three-Dimensional Reconstruction of the Femoral Artery Bifurcation with Non-Invasive B-mode Ultrasound and a New Position Registration Device. J Vasc Technology 1993; 17: 211-216.
29. Patwari P, Carr SC, Vonesh MJ, et al. A novel technique for three-dimensional reconstruction of vascular ultrasound: initial results. J Am Coll Cardiol 1996; 29:125A.
30. Barzalai B, Saffitz JE, Miller JG, Sobel BE. Quantitative ultrasonic characterization of the nature of atherosclerotic plaques in human aorta. Circ Res, 1987; 60:459-463.
31. Ng KH, Vonesh MJ, Garti JT, Morales RE, Roth SI, McPherson DD. Intravascular ultrasonic characterization of atherosclerotic plaques. Circulation, 1993; 88:1-502.
32. New RRC. Preparation of liposomes. In: Liposomes a practical approach. New RRC (ed), Oxford University Press, 1992; 33-104.
33. Unger E, Fritz T, Kulik B, et al. Gas filled lipid bylayers as ultrasound contrast agents. Invest Radiol 1994;29:S134-S136.
34. Alkan-Onyuksel H, Demos SM, Lanza GM, et al. Development of inherently echogenic liposomes as an ultrasonic contrast agent. J Pharm Sci 1996; 85:486-490.
35. Demos SM, Alkan-Onyuksel H, Gilbert J, et al. In-vitro targeting of antibody-conjugated echogenic liposomes for site specific ultrasonic image enhancement. J Pharm Sci 1997; 86:167-171.
36. Berman JW, Calderon TM. The role of endothelial cell adhesion molecules in the development of atherosclerosis. Cardiovascular Path 1992; 1:17-28.
37. O'Brien K, Allen M, McDonald, T. Vascular cell adhesion molecule is expressed in human coronary atherosclerotic plaques: implications for the mode to progression of advanced coronary atherosclerosis. J Clin Invest 1993; 92:945-951.
38. Davis CA, Pearce WH, Haines GK, Shah M, Koch AE . Increased ICAM-1 expression in aortic disease. J Biomech 1993; 19:351-358.
39. Poston R, Haskard DO, Coucher J, Gall NP, Johnson-Tidey R.   Expression of intracellular adhesion molecule-1 in atherosclerotic plaques. Am J Pathol 1992; 140:665-673.
40. Loscalzo J. The relation between atherosclerosis and thrombosis. Circulation 1992; 86:S95-S96.
41. Lanza GM, Wallace KD, Abendschein DA, et al. Acoustic enhancement of arterial thrombi in vivo following intravenous injection. Circulation 1996; 94:I-319.
42. Lanza GM, Fischer SE,, Wallace KD, et al. Three dimensional depiction of thrombus topology imaged with intravascular ultrasound after acoustical enhancement with a specific fibrin targeted ultrasonic contrast agent. Circulation 1996: 94:I-664.
43. McCreery TP, Sweitzer RH, Wu G, et al. Targeted Ultrasound contrast agents for the detection of thrombosis. Circulation 1996: 94:I-664.
44. Evans JL, Ng KH, Vonesh MJ, et al. Arterial imaging utilizing a new forward viewing intravascular ultrasound catheter: initial studies. Circulation 1994; 89:712-717.
45. Wiet SP, Ng KH, Vonesh MJ, et al. Initial in-vivo studies using a new forward viewing intravascular ultrasound catheter. J Am Coll Cardiol 1994; 3:291A.
46. Ng KH, Evans JL, Vonesh MJ, et al. Three dimensional reconstruction and display of forward viewing intravascular ultrasound data. Circulation 1994; 89:718-723.
47. Vonesh MJ, Mockros LF, Davidson CJ, Chandran KB, McPherson DD. Vascular acoustic emission accompany arterial injury and potential applications to balloon angioplasty. Ann Biomed Eng 1997; (In Press).
48. Vonesh MJ, Mockros LF, Chandran KB, Davidson CJ, McPherson DD. In-vitro identification of angioplasty - induced injury using vascular acoustic emissions. Circulation 1997; 95:1022-1029.

POTENTIAL USES FOR ULTRASOUND IMAGING IN CLINICAL TRIALS OF ATHEROMA PROGRESSION AND REGRESSION

Randal J. Thomas, M.D., M.S.

Heart Life Program, Greenville Hospital System
Greenville, South Carolina U.S.A.

Contents

"The quick harvest of pure science is the usable process, the medicine, the machine.
The shy fruit of pure science is understanding."

Lincoln Barnett

I. INTRODUCTION

Important advances have been made in recent years in both the management and evaluation of persons with cardiovascular disease. Several trials have reported that the aggressive management of cardiovascular disease (CVD) risk factors (e.g., dyslipidemia) can halt and even reverse the atherosclerotic process (1-12). The results of these trials have encouraged the adoption of aggressive management guidelines for persons with CVD (13).

While these advances were being developed in the treatment of persons with cardiovascular disease, even more striking advances were taking place in cardiovascular imaging technology. These technological advances have helped clarify our understanding of the origins and sequelae of atherosclerosis and have been reviewed in detail in previous chapters. Despite the rapid speed of these advances, while a tribute to the innovative work among imaging investigators, they have nonetheless raised important questions regarding the usefulness of these new methodologies (14). Do new imaging techniques offer advantages over older techniques? Do they provide new information or rather a different version of "old" information? What is their role in future studies of cardiovascular disease?

To help put these issues into perspective, it is appropriate to first consider the direction in which regression trials are headed. What will be the emphasis of future regression studies? What questions will they attempt to answer? Will ultrasound imaging be an integral part of future studies?.

II. REGRESSION TRIALS: WHERE HAVE WE BEEN?

As depicted in Table 1, studies of CVD regression have evaluated the effects of aggressive risk factor management among select populations, generally either persons with pre-existing CVD or those at very high risk of CVD (e.g., persons with familial hyperlipidemia) (1-10). Most study participants have been middle-aged men, although results in women and in older adults have also been reported (3,5,10). The intervention most commonly studied in most regression trials has been lipid-lowering therapy, although some have included anti-hypertensive therapy (15), antiplatelet therapy (16), and modification of multiple CVD risk factor (6,10).

Given the relatively large number of study participants that would be required to measure changes in mortality and morbidity, most regression trials published to date have studied the effects of risk factor modification on intermediate outcome measures, such as the degree of coronary artery stenosis. More recently, however, trials have found significant improvements in mortality and morbidity (3,4,7). In fact, the differences in mortality and morbidity between treatment and control groups in these trials have been much larger than would have been predicted by the relatively small improvements in the vascular lumen measurements alone. The exact explanation of this observation is unclear, but may be due at least in part to an effect of lipid-lowering therapy on plaque stabilization and improvements in endothelial function, resulting in improvements in coronary perfusion. The question then that still needs to be addressed by future trials with hypolipidemic drugs is the mechanisms whereby they reduce mortality and morbidity. It is likely that cardiovascular imaging will play a crucial role in providing this type of information.

The coronary arteries have been the vascular bed most often studied in atheroma regression trials. The CLAS study did include angiographic analysis of the femoral as well as the coronary arteries, before and after lipid-lowering drug therapy, although evidence for reversal of atherosclerosis was less striking in the femoral compared with the coronary arteries (8). Due to the shortcomings of using coronary angiography to evaluate atheroma regression (i.e., invasive, cannot evaluate underlying atheromatous remodeling, unable to evaluate endothelial changes) other methodologies have been utilized (17-19).

The carotid bed is particularly attractive for evaluating atheroma regression since its atherosclerotic activity is a close surrogate for coronary atherosclerosis (20,21), and since it is easily accessible by non-invasive ultrasound, allowing repeated, low-risk evaluations of atheroma regression. In addition, for cerebrovascular disease it is the bed most often associated with occlusive and embolic stroke (21). Recent trials have included the analysis of the carotid arteries and have found that lipid-lowering therapy promotes beneficial changes in carotid atherosclerosis as well as a reduction in cardiac events (i.e., fatal and non-fatal myocardial infarction) (11,12). This correlation between carotid and coronary atherosclerosis has been suggested in previous studies and is supported by epidemiologic evidence that the known risk factors for coronary atherosclerosis are the same as those for carotid atherosclerosis (20,21).

Finally, previous regression trials have used angiography as the imaging method of choice with the exception of recent studies which have also included ultrasound imaging of the peripheral arteries (11,12,22). The advantages and limitations to both angiography and ultrasonography have been discussed in previous a chapter (see Chapter--Mercuri).

III.   REGRESSION TRIALS: WHERE ARE WE HEADED?

The forces that will shape the future direction of atherosclerosis regression trials are complex and involve an interplay between advances in medicine, the needs of society, and availability of resources. It is apparent that the latter will be an increasingly important factor for the future of biomedical research. Large scale, expensive, and long-term studies involving high risk procedures and treatments will find funding to be scarce, when compared with smaller, less expensive, and short-term studies in which the risks to participants are minimal. With this in mind, where will regression trials be headed in the near future?

Numerous important issues will be at the forefront in future studies of atheroma regression (Table 1). Some of these issues revolve around the testing of new imaging and treatment strategies. Still others issues revolve around the confirmation of previous regression studies in new patient populations or settings. Several of these issues are outlined below:

A. Which Patients Will Be Studied?

Studies are in progress that will assess the possibility of atheroma regression among post-menopausal women with documented CVD. Although the process of atherosclerosis is similar for women and men, there are sex-related differences in the timing of CVD (i.e., women tend to develop atherosclerosis later than men) and the risk factors for CVD (e.g., estrogen deficiency is a risk factor in women, but not in men, and diabetes appears to be a stronger risk factor for women than for men). These differences suggest the need for specific regression trials among women (23).

The same might be argued regarding trials of atheroma regression among the rarely

Table 1. *Past trends and future expectations for atheroma regression trials*

	PAST TRENDS	FUTURE EXPECTATIONS
PATIENT POPULATION	Select groups of mostly high risk, middle-aged, caucasian men	More generalized groups with broader risk and age ranges men and women caucasians and minorities
TREATMENTS	Principally lipid-lowering drug therapy; Rarely, studies involving calcium channel antagonists, and multiple risk factor modification	New lipid-lowering therapies anti-hypertensive therapies anti-diabetes therapies smoking cessation, exercise anti-thrombotic therapy gene therapy smooth muscle regulators endothelial cell regulator fibrinogen regulators
VASCULAR BEDS STUDIED	Principally coronary arteries; rarely studies involving femoral and carotid arteries	Coronary arteries will remain important; carotid artery may become primary study site
OUTCOME MEASURES	Principally lumen stenoses; occasional studies involving mortality, morbidity, and intima-media thickness	Principally measures of arterial wall morphology and physiology
IMAGING METHODS	Principally angiography	Principally ultrasonography

studied non-white populations. Current evidence suggests, however, that environmental risk factors for the development of CVD are similar among the white and non-white populations (24). Still, the relative importance of traditional CVD risk factors in the development of CVD may differ between ethnic and racial groups, possibly due to differences in their genetic "resistance" to environmental factors. For instance, rates of CVD among Latinos in the Southwestern United States are lower than for non-Latino whites in the same area, despite the fact that Latinos are more likely than non-Latino whites to have diabetes and obesity, while rates of hypertension, hypercholesterolemia, and smoking are similar (25).

It is likely that studies of atheroma regression will continue to be carried out among populations at high risk of having CVD. To study populations at low risk of atherosclerosis (the young) would be costly and time consuming unless imaging methods are used which are: (1) non-invasive (low-risk and easily repeated), (2) able to measure very early atherosclerotic changes in the arterial wall, and (3) low cost. If such methods can be employed, studies of the reversal of atherogenesis among low risk groups will be feasible.

B. Which Treatments Will Be Studied?

Treatment strategies aimed at correcting dyslipidemias will probably remain in the forefront of atheroma regression trials in the future. Previously successful lipid-lowering drug (statins, resins, and niacin) and diet therapies will be tested against newer management strategies, including antioxidants and novel regulators of lipoprotein metabolism. In addition, drug and non-drug treatments for other traditional CVD risk factors (hypertension, diabetes, smoking, and physical inactivity) as well as non-traditional risk factors (e.g., hyperhomocysteinemia) will be studied as potential reversing agents of atherogenesis. Calcium channel antagonists and ACE inhibitors have been and will continue to be tested in as potential promoters of atheroma regression (15,26). New therapies (e.g., gene therapy, smooth muscle cell regulators, and endothelial cell regulators) will be developed and tested for their anti-atherogenic potential (27). Finally, and perhaps most importantly, the benefits of drug and non-drug interventions for atheroma regression will be tested head-to-head against the benefits of coronary and peripheral artery revascularization procedures.

C. Which Outcomes Will Be Measured?

The exact outcomes to be measured in future regression trials depend upon four inter-related factors: (1) the availability of resources, (2) the development of imaging technology, (3) the effectiveness of therapies under investigation, and (4) the identification of reliable intermediate outcome measures, considered surrogates for morbidity and mortality outcome measures. Certainly, if very limited resources are available for clinical trials it is unlikely that funding will be available for large scale, long-term regression trials designed to detect treatment effects on participant mortality and morbidity rates. Conversely, the identification of more accurate imaging methods, more efficacious treatment regimens, and reliable intermediate outcome measures would enhance the ability of investigators to find treatment differences in future regression trials. Smaller sample sizes and shorter follow-up periods would be needed. It should be remembered, however, that there one danger in using surrogate outcome measures--they will always be imprecise compared with mortality and morbidity endpoints. As **William Farr** (1807-1884) once said, **"The death rate is a fact. Anything beyond this is an inference"**.

Unfortunately, treatments that have normalized surrogate markers for CVD mortality have not always been associated with reductions in CVD death rates in intervention trials (28). In addition, current evidence suggests that changes in lumen diameter serve as only a rough surrogate marker for CVD mortality and morbidity (29).

The outcome measure of choice in the majority of previous regression studies has been the change in lumen characteristics. This will probably continue to be the case for studies concerned mainly with the later stages of atherogenesis (30). There is growing evidence, however, that links atherogenesis--particularly early atherogenesis--with the morphologic and physiologic characteristics of the arterial wall, suggesting that future regression studies will place more and more emphasis on wall characteristics (27). Studies will need to assess the relative speed of atheroma regression and progression in late and early stages of atherogenesis. For instance, if changes in atherosclerosis occur more slowly during early stages of atherogenesis than they do during later stages, regression trials aimed at early atherogenesis would require either longer follow-up periods or more precise measurement methods to detect treatment effects.

The best method to quantify changes in atherosclerotic "load" will also need to be clarified in future regression trials. Are global change scores (e.g., change in mean luminal diameter in selected arterial segments) better correlated with mortality and morbidity than are focal change scores (e.g., changes in individual lesions or segments)? Will the combination of change scores be even better (i.e., changes in arterial wall thickness plus changes in plaque morphology plus changes in blood flow characteristics)?

Other questions remain for future studies, including: Which morphologic and physiologic attributes best correlate with improvements in CVD events? Do different atheroma characteristics (morphologic and physiologic) predict different CVD events (myocardial infarction, stable and unstable angina pectoris, stroke, etc.)? Which method of assessing atheroma regression is most cost-effective? Which intervention methods aimed at inducing atheroma regression are most cost-effective?

D. Which Vascular Bed(s) Will be Studied?

Previous studies of atherogenesis have suggested that while the correlation of carotid and coronary atherogenesis is fairly good, the correlation between femoral and coronary atherogenesis is not particularly good (31). Given that coronary heart disease continues to be a major contributor to CVD morbidity and mortality, it is likely that it will remain the focus--direct or indirect--of future trials. The use of carotid artery imaging will more than likely increase, since the carotid arteries can be imaged by relatively inexpensive, non-invasive imaging methods. A regression trial which includes imaging of both the coronary and carotid arterial beds will shed important light on their responsiveness, respectively, to atheroma regression and progression. It is possible, as has been shown by previous investigations, that regression and progression of atheroma proceed at different rates in different vascular beds (8).

E. Which Imaging Methods Will Be Used?

Non-invasive imaging methods will continue to grow in importance in the assessment of atherogenesis, for numerous reasons, including: (1) their relatively low costs, (2) minimal risk to patients, and (3) convenience of testing and re-testing (32). Consequently, studies involving non-invasive imaging methods are less burdened by certain confounding factors that affect the results of studies using invasive imaging methods. For instance, patients in angiographic trials are a select group of patients who have generally been referred for angiographic evaluation, based on their clinical signs and symptoms. Non-invasive imaging can be safely offered to a relatively non-select group of patients. Both invasive and non-invasive imaging are limited by certain other factors, however, such as misclassification bias, operator error, and interpretation error (33).

The choice of imaging methods for future regression trials depends in large part upon the outcome measures that will be included in such studies. There is growing evidence that arterial wall morphology and physiology may be the critical measures to help better understand the process and clinical manifestations of atheroma progression and regression. If such is the case, imaging methods which can assess arterial wall characteristics, such as carotid ultrasound and intravascular ultrasound, will become the preferred imaging method in future regression trials. Given the invasive nature of intravascular ultrasound it is unlikely to be as widely applicable in clinical trials as carotid ultrasound. Carotid ultrasound imaging, in fact, may be the imaging method of choice for regression trials in the future (34).

IV. POTENTIAL ROLE OF NON-INVASIVE ULTRASOUND IMAGING IN REGRESSION TRIALS

As summarized in the previous sections of this chapter, non-invasive ultrasound imaging will continue to assume a role of great importance in monitoring the progression and regression of atherosclerosis in future clinical trials. Future trials, in fact, will need to include surrogate markers for CVD mortality and morbidity, will need to have relatively short follow-up periods, relatively small sample sizes, and relatively low costs per evaluation unit.

Ultrasound imaging of the carotid artery can be applied in a wide variety of patient populations, with relative ease, with minimal risk to the patient, and at relatively low cost. It provides accurate data on important intermediate outcome measures, such as arterial wall morphologic and physiologic characteristics. Although non-invasive ultrasound imaging cannot image the coronary arteries directly, it will still have great utility in studies of atheroma regression since atherogenesis in the carotid arteries is correlated with atherogenic activity of the coronary arteries (32). All of these factors place ultrasound imaging in a very promising position for future regression studies.

Will ultrasound imaging be able to expand our understanding of atherogenesis or simply expand our databases with similar information to that which has already been reported in angiographic trials? Several lines of investigation involving ultrasound imaging have the potential for adding new and important data on the atherogenic process, studies of arterial wall thickness, plaque morphology and content, vasomotion, and blood flow characteristics, as described below.

A. Arterial Wall Thickness

Ultrasound assessment of arterial wall thickness has already added important new information to our understanding of atheroma progression and regression. There is evidence, for example, that intima-media thickness (IMT) of the carotid artery serves as an accurate surrogate measure for CVD morbidity and mortality. Previous studies have shown, for example, that IMT correlates with risk of CVD events (32) and more recent studies suggest that lipid-lowering therapy can reduce IMT and subsequent CVD events (11,12). It is clear that mean or composite measures of IMT are more accurate and precise than are single measures. It is still unclear, however, if mean measures of IMT are more accurate than single or maximal measures in predicting clinical CVD events at the individual patient level.

Measurement of IMT helps reduce the confounding effect of arterial remodeling that adversely affects the accuracy of angiographic measurements of luminal stenoses. On the other hand, data have not yet been published which show IMT to be as good or better at predicting CVD events as angiographic measurements of luminal stenoses. Newer techniques such as three-dimensional reconstruction of the carotid artery with B-mode ultrasound (as addressed in the previous chapter) may allow for complementary quantification of plaque load with standard IMT measurements.

B. Plaque Characteristics

An emerging role for ultrasound imaging is in the quantification and characterization of the atherosclerotic lesion itself. Clearly, there are technical difficulties in the accurate visualization of certain plaque characteristics (i.e., fibrous caps and ulceration)(32,33). Technological advances in this area, however, will continue to enhance the technical abilities of ultrasound to image atheroma, as described in earlier chapters (e.g., three-dimensional visualization of plaque, radiofrequency tissue characterization, and acoustic enhancement of atheroma components). This should open up numerous issues for potentially fruitful investigation, including:

1. Do beneficial changes in plaque morphology occur with CVD risk factor modification?
2. Do these changes predict improvements in clinical manifestations of atherosclerosis?
3. Does CVD risk factor modification produce changes in plaque morphology or plaque content or both? Which is more important clinically?
4. Does plaque instability and disruption occur less often in the setting of atheroma regression?

C. Endothelial Dysfunction

There is evidence that disorders of coronary vasomotion and the development of arterial stiffness are associated with the development of atherosclerosis (35,36). There is some evidence, in fact , to suggest that endothelial dysfunction may be one of the first steps in the process of atherogenesis (37). Thus, ultrasound imaging of endothelial function will be particularly helpful in illuminating the relationship between early atherogenesis, treatment of CVD risk factors, and clinically manifest CVD events.

D.   Blood Flow Characteristics

While routine two-dimensional ultrasound imaging of the carotid artery lumen is generally less accurate than angiographic imaging, particularly for severely stenotic arteries, characterization of blood flow patterns (e.g., velocity profiling and shear stress estimates by Doppler ultrasound) appear to be accurate physiologic reflections of the arterial lumen (38). Studies are needed that can assess questions such as:

1. Are blood flow patterns more sensitive to atheroma regression than are angiographic measurements of luminal stenoses?
2. Are changes in blood flow patterns with atheroma regression better predictors of clinical events than are angiographic findings?
3. Are blood flow characteristics in the carotid arteries related to those in the coronary arteries?

V. Summary

There have been impressive advances in the past two decades in the clinical management of patients with atherosclerosis and the visualization of atherogenic process itself. Previous clinical trials have identified treatments which can promote the regression of coronary and carotid atherosclerosis. Visualization of this regression has traditionally relied upon angiographic measurement of luminal stenoses, although recent studies have documented carotid artery regression using B-mode ultrasound.

Regression trials will continue to play a prominent role in the near future, although such trials will of necessity need to minimize costs, sample sizes and follow-up time while still maintaining sufficient power to ascertain appropriate outcome measures. Surrogate outcome measures will be used commonly as long as they can be closely correlated with mortality and morbidity. Regression trials will need to be expanded to new patient populations and will involve an expanding array of treatment modalities. Ultrasound imaging of the carotid artery may be the imaging method of choice for future studies of atheroma control, particularly in studies of early atherosclerosis. The exact role of directly imaging of the coronary arteries by invasive methods will depend directly on the accuracy of non-invasive methods (e.g., B-mode ultrasound) to predict coronary heart disease outcomes. Ultrasound imaging holds great promise in measuring arterial wall thickness, atheroma morphology and content, vasomotion, and blood flow characteristics which may result in the more precise and multidimensional assessment of atheroma progression and regression in the future.

References

1. Brensike JF, Levy RI, Kelsey SF, et al. Effects of therapy with cholestyramine on progression of coronary arteriosclerosis: results of the NHLBI Type II Coronary Intervention Study. Circulation 1984; 69:313-24.
2. Blankenhorn DH, Nessim SA, Johnson RL, et al. Beneficial effects of combined colestipol-niacin therapy on coronary atherosclerosis and coronary venous bypass grafts. JAMA 1987; 257:3233-40.
3. Scandinavian Simvastatin Survival Study Group. Randomized trial of cholesterol lowering in 4444 patients with coronary heart disease: the Scandinavian Simvastatin Survival Study (4S). Lancet 1994; 344:1383-9.
4. Shepherd J, Cobbe SM, Ford I, et al. for the West of Scotland Coronary Prevention Study Group. Prevention of coronary heart disease with pravastatin in men with hypercholesterolemia. N Engl J Med. 1995 ; 333:1301-7.
5. Kane JP, Malloy MJ, Ports TA, et al. Regression of coronary atherosclerosis during treatment of familial hypercholesterolemia with combined drug regimens. JAMA 1990; 264:3007-3012.
6. Ornish D, Brown SE, Scherwitz LW, et al. Can lifestyle changes reverse coronary heart disease? The Lifestyle Heart Trial. Lancet 1990; 336:129-133.
7. Sacks FM, Pfeffer MA, Moye LA, et al. for the Cholesterol and Recurrent Events Trial Investigators. The effect of pravastatin on coronary events after myocardial infarction in patients with average cholesterol levels. N Engl J Med 1996; 335:1001-9.

8.   Blankenhorn DH, Azen SP, Crawford DW, et al. Effects of colestipol-niacin therapy on human femoral atherosclerosis. Circulation 1991; 83:438-47.
9.   Blankenhorn DH, Azen SP, Kramsch DM, et al. Coronary angiographic changes with lovastatin therapy. The Monitored Atherosclerosis Regression Study (MARS). Ann Intern Med 1993; 119:969-76.
10. Haskell WL, Alderman EL, Fair JM, et al. Effects of intensive multiple risk factor reduction on coronary atherosclerosis and clinical cardiac events in men and women with coronary artery disease. The Stanford Coronary Risk Intervention Project (SCRIP). Circulation 1994; 89:975-90.
11. Crouse III JR, Byington RP, Bond MG, et al. Pravastatin, lipids, and atherosclerosis in the carotid arteries (PLAC-II). Am J Cardiol 1995; 75:455-9.
12. Furberg CD, Adams HP, Applegate WB, et al. Effect of lovastatin on early carotid atherosclerosis and cardiovascular events. Circulation 1994; 90:1679-87.
13. Expert Panel on Detection, Evaluation, and Treatment of High Blood Cholesterol in Adults. Summary of the second report of the National Cholesterol Education Program (NCEP) expert panel on detection, evaluation, and treatment of high blood cholesterol in adults (Adult Treatment Panel II). JAMA 1993; 269:3015-23.
14. Kuller LH. AHA symposium/epidemiology meeting: Atherosclerosis. Discussion: Why measure atherosclerosis? Circulation (suppl II):II-34-II-37.
15. Waters DW, Lesperance J, Francetich M, et al. A controlled clinical trial to assess the effect of a calcium channel blocker on the progression of coronary atherosclerosis. Circulation 1990; 82:1940-1953.
16. Chesebro JH, Webster MWI, Smith HC, et al. Anti-platelet therapy in coronary disease progression: Reduced infarction and new lesion formation. Circulation 1989; 80:II-266.
17. McPherson DD, Sirna SJ, Hiratzka LF, et al. Coronary arterial remodeling studied by high-frequency epicardial echocardiography: an early compensatory mechanism in patients with obstructive coronary atherosclerosis. J Am Coll Cardiol 1991; 17:79-86.
18. Glagov S, Weisenberg E, Zarins DK, et al. Compensatory enlargement of human atherosclerotic coronary arteries. N Engl J Med 1987; 316:1371-5.
19. McPherson DD, Hiratzka LF, Lamberth WC, et al. Delineation of the extent of coronary atherosclerosis by high-frequency epicardial echocardiography. N Engl J Med 1987; 316:304-9.
20. Craven TE, Ryu JE, Espeland MA, et al. Evaluation of the association between carotid artery atherosclerosis and coronary artery stenosis: a case-comparison study. Circulation 1990; 82:1230-42.
21. Heiss G, Sharrett AR, Barnes R, et al. Carotid atherosclerosis measured by B-mode ultrasound in populations: associations with cardiovascular risk factors in the ARIC study. Am J Epidemiol 1991; 134:250-6.
22. Mack WJ, Selzer RH, Hodis HN, et al. One-year reduction and longitudinal analysis of carotid intima-media thickness associated with colestipol/niacin therapy. Stroke 1993; 24:1779-83.
23. Wenger NK, Speroff L, Packard B. Cardiovascular health and disease in women. N Engl J Med 1993; 329:247-56.
24. AHA Medical/Scientific Statement. Special report. Cardiovascular diseases and stroke in African-Americans and other racial minorities in the United States. A statement for health professionals. Circulation 1991; 83:1462-80.
25. Mitchell BD, Hazuda HP, Haffner SM, et al. Myocardial infarction in Mexican-Americans and non-Hispanic whites. The San Antonio Heart Study. Circulation 1991; 83:45-51.
26. Borhani NO, Mercuri M, Borhani PA, et al. Final outcome results of the Multicenter Isradipine Diuretic Atherosclerosis Study (MIDAS). A randomized controlled trial. JAMA 1996; 276:785-91.
27. Schwartz CJ, Valente AJ, Sprague EA, et al. Atherosclerosis. Potential targets for stabilization and regression. Circulation 1992; 86(suppl III):III-117-III-123.
28. Cardiac Arrhythmia Suppression Trial (CAST): Special report: Effect of encainide and flecainide on mortality in a randomized trial of arrhythmia suppression after myocardial infarction. N Engl J Med 1989; 321:406-12.
29. Buchwald H, Matts JP, Fitch LL, et al. Changes in sequential coronary arteriograms and subsequent coronary events. JAMA 1992; 268:1429-33.
30. Crouse JR, Thompson CJ. An evaluation of methods for imaging and quantifying coronary and carotid lumen stenosis and atherosclerosis. Circulation 1993; 87(suppl II):II-17-II-33.
31. Salonen JT, Salonen R. Ultrasound B-mode imaging in observational studies of atherosclerotic progression. Circulation 1993; 87(suppl II):II-56-II-65.
32. Probstfield JL, Byington RP, Egan DA, et al. Methodological issues facing studies of atherosclerotic change. Circulation 1993; 87(suppl II):II-74-II-81.
33. Sharrett AR. Invasive versus noninvasive studies of risk factors and atherosclerosis. Circulation 1993; 87(suppl II):II-48-II-53.

34. Cashin-Hemphill L. Femoral and coronary angiographic trials. Am J Cardiol 1993; 71:20B-25B.
35. Zeiver AM, Schachinger V, Saurbier B, Just H. Assessment of endothelial modulation of coronary vasomotor tone: insights into a fundamental functional disturbance in vascular biology of atherosclerosis. Basic Research in Cardiology. 1994; 89 (suppl 1):115-28.
36. Zeiver AM, Schachlinger V, Hohnloser SH, et al. Coronary atherosclerotic wall thickening and vascular reactivity in humans. Elevated high-density lipoprotein levels ameliorate abnormal vasoconstriction in early atherosclerosis. Circulation 1994; 89:2525-32.
37. Reddy KG, Nair RN, Sheehan HM, Hodgson JM. Evidence that selective endothelial dysfunction may occur in the absence of angiographic or ultrasound atherosclerosis in patients with risk factors for atherosclerosis. J Am Coll Cardiol 1994; 23:833-43.
38. Blakeley DD, Oddone EZ, Hasselblad V, et al. Noninvasive carotid artery testing. A meta-analytic review. Ann Intern Med 1995; 122:360-7.

INDEX